Advances in Movement Disorders

Indian Academy of Neurology

Advances in Movement Disorders

Editor-in-Chief

Debashish Chowdhury
DTCD MD(Medicine) DM(Neurology) FIAN FRCP(Edinburgh)
Commonwealth Fellow in Stroke Medicine(Edinburgh)
Director–Professor and Head
Department of Neurology
GB Pant Institute of Postgraduate Medical Education and Research
New Delhi, India

Editors

U Meenakshisundaram MD DM
FAAN FIAN FRCP FPRD FMDSI
Director and Senior Consultant
Neurologist
MGM Healthcare
Chennai, Tamil Nadu, India

Achal Kumar Srivastava MD DM
Professor
Department of Neurology
All India Institute of Medical Sciences
New Delhi, India

Associate Editors

Roopa Rajan MD DM
Additional Professor
Department of Neurology
All India Institute of Medical
Sciences
New Delhi, India

Divyani Garg MD DM
Assistant Professor
Department of Neurology
All India Institute of Medical
Sciences
New Delhi, India

Sreenivas UM MD DM MRCP
SCE FEBN
Consultant Neurologist
Department of Neurology
MGM Healthcare
Chennai, Tamil Nadu, India

Foreword

Kailash Bhatia

JAYPEE

JAYPEE BROTHERS MEDICAL PUBLISHERS
The Health Sciences Publisher
New Delhi | London

Jaypee Brothers Medical Publishers (P) Ltd

Headquarters
EMCA House
23/23-B, Ansari Road, Daryaganj
New Delhi 110 002, India
Landline: +91-11-23272143, +91-11-23272703
+91-11-23282021, +91-11-23245672
E-mail: jaypee@jaypeebrothers.com

Corporate Office
Jaypee Brothers Medical Publishers (P) Ltd.
4838/24, Ansari Road, Daryaganj
New Delhi 110 002, India
Phone: +91-11-43574357
Fax: +91-11-43574314
E-mail: jaypee@jaypeebrothers.com

Overseas Office
JP Medical Ltd.
83, Victoria Street, London
SW1H 0HW (UK)
Phone: +44-20 3170 8910
E-mail: info@jpmedpub.com

EU GPSR Authorised Representative
Logos Europe, 9 rue Nicolas Poussin
17000, La Rochelle, France
Phone: +33 (0) 6 67 93 73 78
E-mail: Contact@logoseurope.eu

Website: www.jaypeebrothers.com
Website: www.jaypeedigital.com

Inquiries for bulk sales may be solicited at: jaypee@jaypeebrothers.com

IAN Advances in Movement Disorders / ***Debashish Chowdhury, U Meenakshisundaram, Achal Kumar Srivastava***

First Edition: 2025, Reprint 2025

ISBN: 978-93-6616-794-7

Printed in India

Indian Academy of Neurology

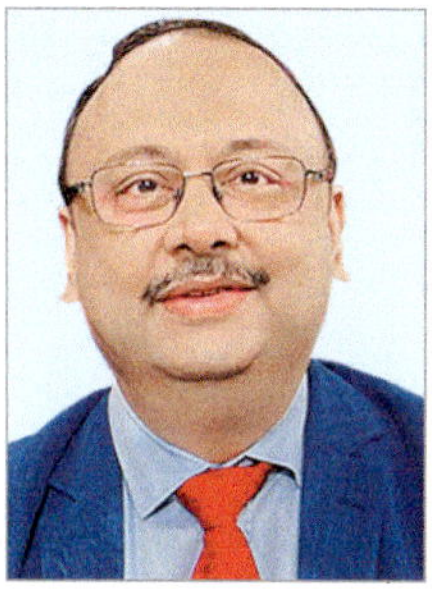

PRESIDENT
Debashish Chowdhury
New Delhi, India

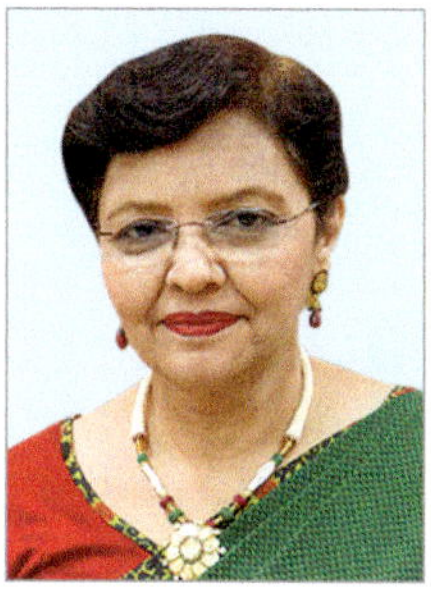

PRESIDENT-ELECT
Sangeeta Ravat
Mumbai, Maharashtra, India

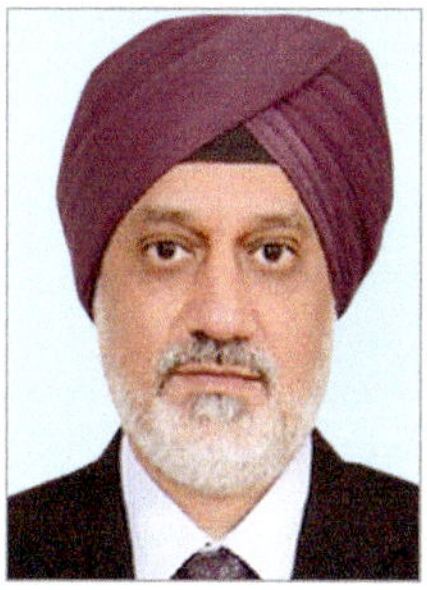

IMMEDIATE PAST PRESIDENT
Gagandeep Singh
Ludhiana, Punjab, India

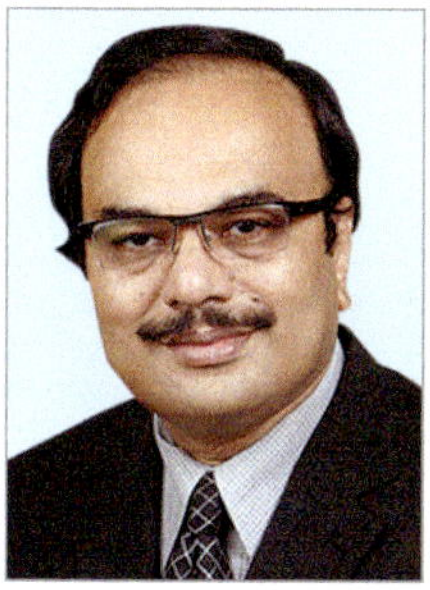

PAST PRESIDENT
Nirmal Surya
Mumbai, Maharashtra, India

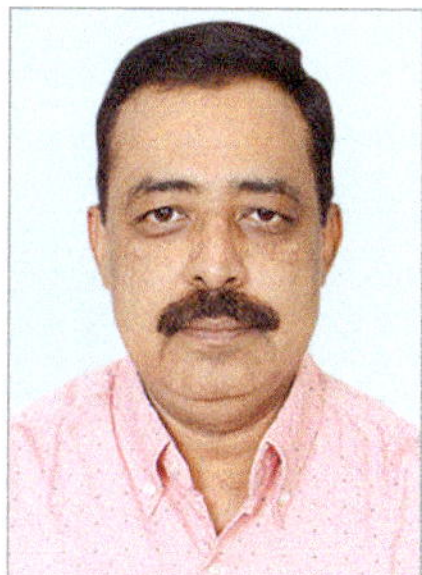

TREASURER
Achal Srivastava
New Delhi, India

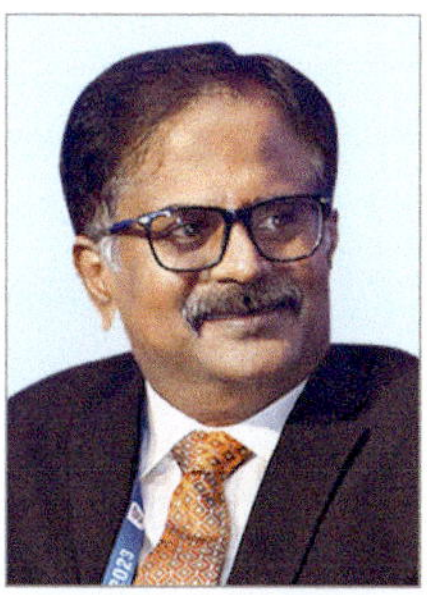

SECRETARY
U Meenakshisundaram
Chennai, Tamil Nadu, India

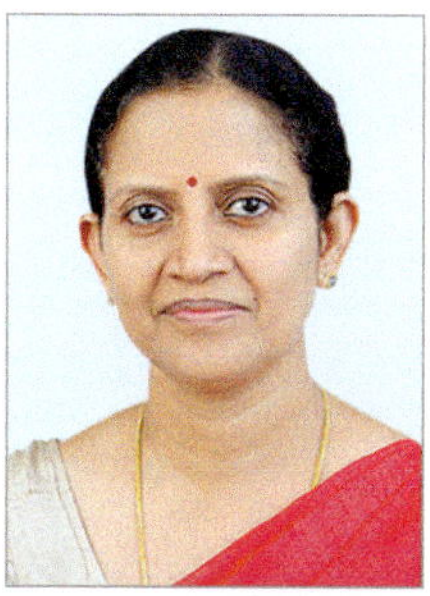

EDITOR, ANNALS OF IAN
PN Sylaja
Thiruvananthapuram, Kerala, India

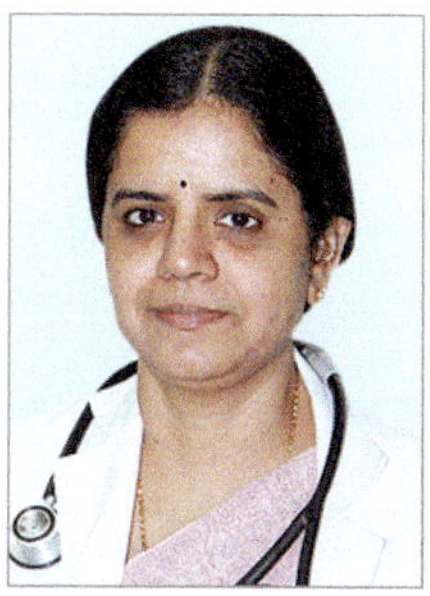

CME CONVENER
Sita Jayalakshmi
Hyderabad, Telangana, India

Executive Members

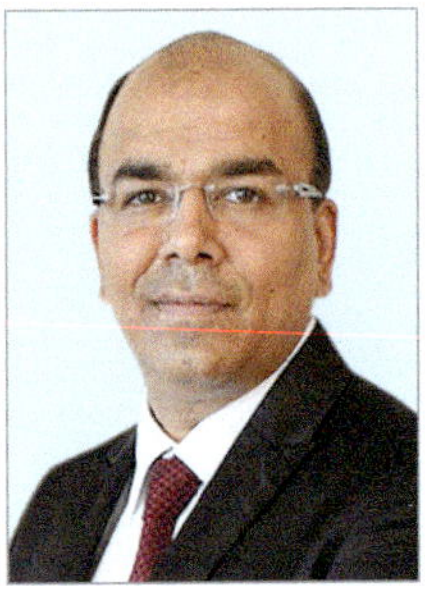

Arvind Sharma
Ahmedabad, Gujarat, India

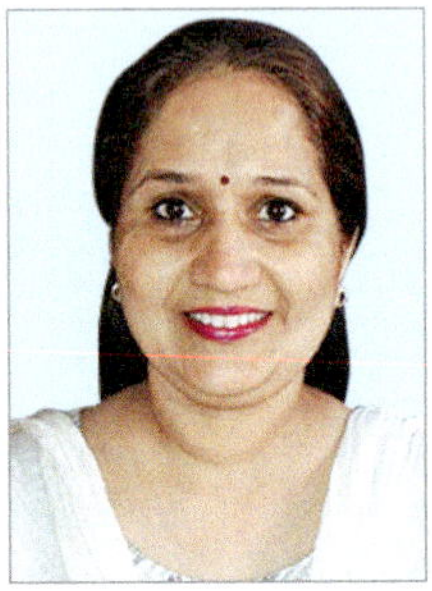

Bhawna Sharma
Jaipur, Rajasthan, India

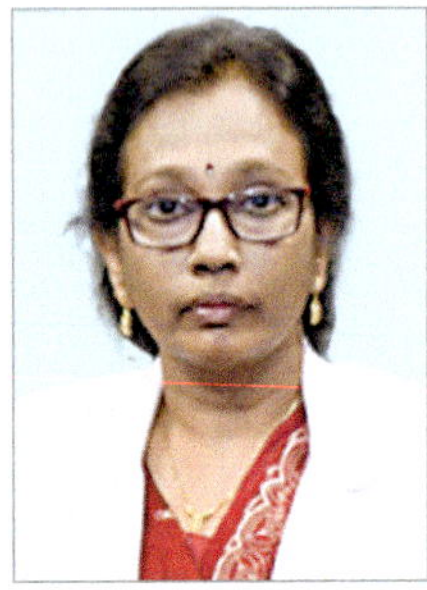

Atchayaram Nalini
Bengaluru, Karnataka, India

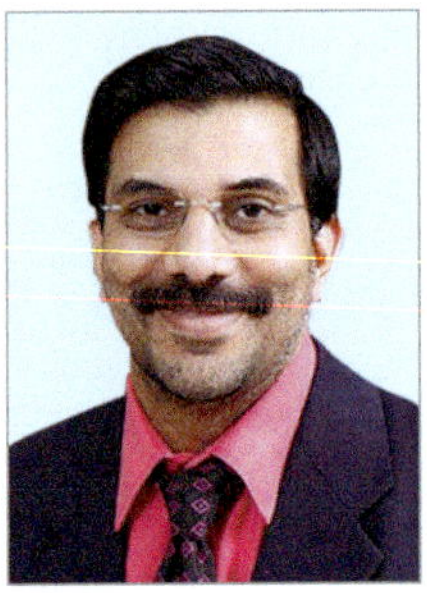

JOINT TREASURER
Pradeep VG
Kozhikode, Kerala, India

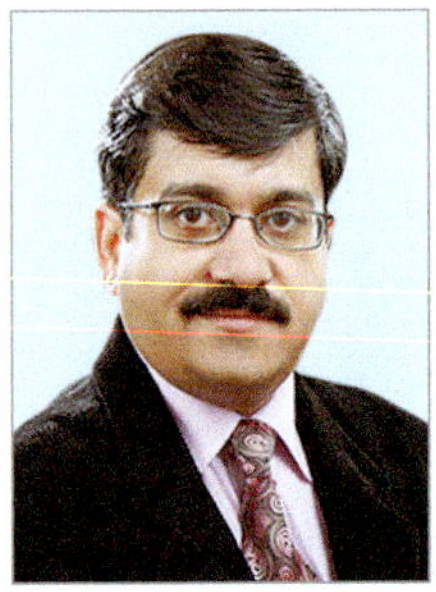

JOINT SECRETARY
Sumit Singh
Gurugram, Haryana, India

Contributors

Abhishek Vaingankar MD
Senior Resident
Department of Neurology
All India Institute of Medical Sciences
New Delhi, India

Achal Kumar Srivastava MD DM
Professor
Department of Neurology
All India Institute of Medical Sciences
New Delhi, India

Asha Kishore MD DM FRCP
Director
Movement Disorders Centre
Aster Medcity
Kochi, Kerala, India

Asish Vijayaraghavan MD DM PDF(Movement Disorders)
Assistant Professor
Comprehensive Care Centre for Movement Disorders
Department of Neurology
Sree Chitra Tirunal Institute for Medical Sciences and Technology
Thiruvananthapuram, Kerala, India

Ayush Agarwal MD DM
Assistant Professor
Department of Neurology
All India Institute of Medical Sciences
New Delhi, India

Divya Kalikavil Puthanveedu MD DM
Additional Professor
Comprehensive Care Centre for Movement Disorders
Department of Neurology
Sree Chitra Tirunal Institute for Medical Sciences and Technology
Thiruvananthapuram, Kerala, India

Divya M Radhakrishnan MD DM
Associate Professor
Department of Neurology
All India Institute of Medical Sciences
New Delhi, India

Divyani Garg MD DM
Assistant Professor
Department of Neurology
All India Institute of Medical Sciences
New Delhi, India

G Balaji MD DM
Assistant Professor
Department of Neurology
Chengalpattu Medical College
Chengalpattu, Tamil Nadu, India

Hrishikesh Kumar MD DM PDF
Head, Department of Neurology
Director, Movement Disorder Program
Institute of Neurosciences
Kolkata, West Bengal, India

Jacky Ganguly MD DM PDF
Consultant
Movement Disorder Centre
Institute of Neurosciences
Kolkata, West Bengal, India

Karthik Harisankar DM
Senior Resident
Department of Neurology
PGIMER
Chandigarh, India

Kartika Gulati DM
Clinical Fellow
Department of Neurology and Stroke Medicine
Amrita Hospital
Faridabad, Haryana, India

Kuldeep Shetty DM
Consultant Neurologist
Department of Neurology
Mazumdar Shaw Medical Center
Narayana Health City
Bengaluru, Karnataka, India

Lakshmanan S DM
Consultant Neurologist
Department of Neurology
Kauvery Hospital
Chennai, Tamil Nadu, India

Manu SG MD DM
PDF Movement Disorders
Department of Neurology
Parkinson's and Movement Disorders Centre
Aster Medcity
Kochi, Kerala, India

Pramod Kumar Pal MD DNB DM FIAN FRCP
Professor
Department of Neuroimaging and Interventional Radiology
Department of Neurology
National Institute of Mental Health and Neurosciences (NIMHANS)
Bengaluru, Karnataka, India

Prashanth LK DM
Consultant Movement Disorder Specialist
Department of Neurology
Parkinson's Disease and Movement Disorders Clinic
Bengaluru, Karnataka, India

P Vijayashankar MD DM
Consultant Neurologist
Department of Neurology
Apollo Hospitals
Greams Road, Chennai, Tamil Nadu, India

Ravi Yadav MD DM
Professor
Department of Neurology
National Institute of Mental Health and Neurosciences (NIMHANS)
Bengaluru, Karnataka, India

Roopa Rajan MD DM
Additional Professor
Department of Neurology
All India Institute of Medical Sciences
New Delhi, India

Sahil Mehta DM
Additional Professor
Department of Neurology
PGIMER
Chandigarh, India

Samim MM MD DM
Senior Resident
Department of Neurology
National Institute of Mental Health and Neurosciences (NIMHANS)
Bengaluru, Karnataka, India

Sampurna Chowdhury MD
Senior Resident
Department of Neurology
All India Institute of Medical Sciences
New Delhi, India

Sanjay Pandey DM
Professor and Head
Department of Neurology and Stroke Medicine, Amrita Hospital
Faridabad, Haryana, India

Sayooja Sachithanandan MD DM
Postdoctoral Fellow in Movement Disorders
Comprehensive Care Centre for Movement Disorders
Department of Neurology
Sree Chitra Tirunal Institute for Medical Sciences and Technology
Thiruvananthapuram, Kerala, India

Shiny Joy MD
Senior Resident
Department of Neurology
All India Institute of Medical Sciences
New Delhi, India

Shweta Prasad MBBS PhD
Welcome DBT Fellow
Department of Neuroimaging and Interventional Radiology
Department of Neurology
National Institute of Mental Health and Neurosciences (NIMHANS)
Bengaluru, Karnataka, India

S Sidharth MD
Senior Resident
Department of Neurology
All India Institute of Medical Sciences
New Delhi, India

Sreenivas UM MD DM MRCP SCE FEBN
Consultant Neurologist
Department of Neurology
MGM Healthcare
Chennai, Tamil Nadu, India

Supriyo Choudhury MD PhD
Consultant Clinical Pharmacologist
Assistant Director of Research
Institute of Neurosciences
Kolkata, West Bengal, India

Syam Krishnan MD DM
Professor
Comprehensive Care Centre for Movement Disorders
Department of Neurology
Sree Chitra Tirunal Institute for Medical Sciences and Technology
Thiruvananthapuram, Kerala, India

U Meenakshisundaram MD DM FAAN FIAN FRCP FPRD FMDSI
Director and Senior Consultant Neurologist
MGM Healthcare
Chennai, Tamil Nadu, India

Vishwakiran Jhawar MD
Senior Resident
Department of Neurology
Mazumdar Shaw Medical Center
Narayana Health City
Bengaluru, Karnataka, India

Foreword

I have watched with great pleasure the advancement of the Indian Academy of Neurology and in particular the Movement Disorders subsection, which has blossomed over the last 12 years and led to experts in the field being recognized not just nationally but also internationally. It is, therefore, befitting that a volume of this form related to the current advances in the management of movement disorders should be put together by these colleagues. This is an impressive volume with contributions from both the seniors such as Professors Pramod Kumar Pal, Asha Kishore, Achal Kumar Srivastava, Hrishikesh Kumar, U Meenakshisundaram, and Sanjay Pandey (and others) and the upcoming stars in the field including Sahil Mehta, Divyani Garg, Ravi Yadav, and others. The focus of the book is management which will be a great boon and a reference source not only for the general neurologists but also for the movement disorders fraternity. The book covers a range of topics including the treatments of early and late Parkinson's disease, dystonia, and drug-induced movement disorders, the latter being quite common in the Indian scenario. Also, a dedicated chapter to Wilsons' disease and its management by Dr Prashanth Kukkle is welcome, as this is very common in India. There are practical chapters on the use of botulinum toxin in movement disorders and the management of tremor, restless legs, and hyperkinetic movement disorders. The chapters on autoimmune movement disorders and their management and emergency room movement disorders are both excellent and will be a valuable reference for all when faced with such a patient. I am sure that this book will be seen for reference in the clinics of most neurology practitioners and for those involved in movement disorders training and also more experienced exponents of the art of movement disorders. My congratulations go to all the authors for putting together this masterpiece.

Kailash Bhatia DM FRCP FEAN
Professor of Clinical Neurology
Department of Clinical and Movement Neuroscience
Institute of Neurology
Queen Square
London, UK

Message from Editor-in-Chief

Dear Readers,

The Indian Academy of Neurology (IAN) has been at the forefront of neurology education and has a rich history of publications which rank high in terms of academic and scientific content. As President, it has been my pleasure to team up with my Executive Committee members, who are experts in various neurological subspecialties and high-quality and prolific authors with an impressive track record of publications, as editors and bring out a series of books which continue to hold high the tradition of IAN in terms of high-impact scientific content.

As Chief Editor of IAN *"Advances in Movement Disorders"*, it is my pleasure to bring to you a book which sets the bar high for content—accurate, updated, and relevant—and at the same time presents it in a reader-friendly manner, which makes the book an ideal companion for everyone interested in the subject. I thank my colleagues and editors of this book, *Dr U Meenakshisundaram and Dr Achal Kumar Srivastava*, for the shared vision of high-quality, focused content as well as excellent support rendered during the making of this book.

This has been our collective effort, and we sincerely hope that each of you will like reading this book as much as we loved bringing this out.

Debashish Chowdhury

Preface

Medicine is an ever-changing exciting science and the information pool keeps morphing at a phenomenal speed. Movement disorders is the fastest growing discipline of neurology where the clinician matters the most, not only in diagnosis but also in making life-changing decisions. Textbooks, especially handy ones like this, are ready reckoners for practical management issues in a busy practice. We sincerely hope that the readers of this book gain updation and satisfaction and, of course, motivation to keep themselves constantly updated.

The expositions in the text focus exclusively on cutting-edge practical management practices. There are 13 chapters and the most important areas of movement disorders for a clinician have been covered. The standard template used in all the chapters will ensure seamless learning and retention.

Publishing a book of this caliber with such a galaxy of experts requires challenging coordination, but all the authors responded enthusiastically and we would like to thank them heartily. The three meticulous associate editors Drs Roopa Rajan, Divyani Garg, and Sreenivas UM deserve much praise for their hard work and dedication. We thank Mr Jitendar Pal Vij (Group Chairman) of Jaypee Brothers Medical Publishers and the entire production team, including Ms Chetna Malhotra (Senior Director—Professional Publishing, Marketing and Business Development) and Mr Prashant Mahajan (Development Editor), for their professional and precise guidance and work.

We are sure that the book will be a valuable addition to already existing books in neurology with the unique feature of being contributed to by neuroscientists of India who have extensive experience in the field of movement disorders.

Debashish Chowdhury
U Meenakshisundaram
Achal Kumar Srivastava

Contents

CHAPTER

1

Current Medical Management of Early Parkinson's Disease

Shweta Prasad, Pramod Kumar Pal

ABSTRACT

Early Parkinson's disease (PD) refers to the initial clinical stage of PD, i.e., <3–5 years of illness, when motor symptoms may not very severe. In contrast to management of later stages of PD, the approach to early PD may need to be highly individualized and requires accounting for numerous factors unrelated to motor symptoms such as the age of the patient, non-motor symptoms (NMS), side-effect profiles and socioeconomic considerations.

Keywords: Early Parkinson's disease, Levodopa, Dopamine agonist.

INTRODUCTION

The term "early Parkinson's disease (PD)" is associated with the stage and duration of the illness, and is unrelated to the age at onset of symptoms. At present, there is no fixed definition of early PD, and this may be attributable to several factors such as which symptom to consider, i.e., motor or non-motor, and the lack of specific diagnostic biomarkers. Although non-motor symptoms (NMS) predate motor symptoms, and current working definitions of early PD are related to the onset of motor symptoms. These include—duration of motor symptoms <3-5 years,[1-3] Hoehn and Yahr (H&Y) stage up to 2.[1,4,5] Often patients may be considered to be early PD, if their symptoms are not severe enough to require dopaminergic treatment,[2,6] or occasionally until the onset of motor complications.[7]

Early PD has been proposed to be classified into preclinical, prodromal, and clinical stages,[8] with the clinical stage being the prime stage for therapeutic intervention. The treatment approach to PD is primarily symptomatic with the eventual aim being reduction in motor disability and improvement of quality of life. Achieving the latter requires additional attention toward the management of NMS. Medical management of early PD is often subject to clinical equipoise.[9] The fundamental debate surrounds the initiation of medical management, i.e., delaying treatment if the motor symptoms are mild, not impairing occupation or lifestyle, or are on the nondominant side of the body—the "wait-and-watch" strategy,[10] or initiation of pharmacotherapy as soon as the diagnosis is made.[11] Proponents for early treatment support the possibility that early dopaminergic treatment may aid in restoration of basal ganglia physiology, leading to a delay in the irreversible modification of circuity.[11,12] While the favor of delaying treatment is based on protection of the patient from inevitable side effects of medication, particularly levodopa associated motor complications.[10,13]

It is imperative to understand that medical management in early PD has to be highly individualized, with significant variance in the approach based on the age of the patient, employment-related implications, lifestyle, NMS, side-effect profile, etc. This chapter reviews the fundamental concepts related to management of motor and NMS of early PD—the main drugs for management, i.e., the well-established approach, newer drugs under evaluation, and recent disease-modifying therapies.

BOX 1: Factors influencing choice of treatment in early Parkinson's disease.

- Age of the patient
- Current occupation
- Symptomatology—motor and nonmotor
- Functional impact of symptoms
- Financial status: Ability to afford medication
- Expectations from treatment: Quick relief versus patience to wait
- Side effect profile of medication
- Coexistent systemic illness

BOX 2: Practical considerations and guidelines for management of early Parkinson's disease.

- Establish whether treatment is needed
- Understand that significant variations exist in the impact of symptoms on a patient's quality of life
- Choice of initiation of treatment and choice of medication should be influenced by the type of symptoms, occupation of the patient, and benefit to adverse effect ratio
- Decisions should involve patients and the caregiver with a flexible and practical approach
- The possibility of fluctuations in symptoms and response to medication should be explained
- Patients should be explained and permitted to modify dosing based on the obtained response
- Credence should be paid to reports of adverse effects, even if minor, and changes should be made accordingly
- The significance of regular and timely consumption of medication and routine follow-up must be emphasized

APPROACH TO MEDICAL MANAGEMENT OF EARLY PARKINSON'S DISEASE

The first step prior to initiation of treatment is to ensure that the patient has early PD. This may occasionally not be clinically obvious owing to the subtle and nonspecific nature of motor symptoms. There are no disease-specific biomarkers for PD, however, it is prudent to rule out other causes of parkinsonism. For instance, imaging plays a significant role particularly in ruling out structural causes of parkinsonism. Awareness of the genotype in case of a genetic variant of PD is helpful in planning therapy as certain genetic subtypes such as *Parkin, PINK1,* and *DJ1* are more likely to develop drug-induced dyskinesias early in the course of illness. The approach to management of early PD extends beyond the status of motor symptoms **(Box 1)** and requires specific considerations **(Box 2)**. Recording a detailed history with focus on the current NMS, non-PD symptoms, comorbidities, and non-PD medication history is crucial. This is particularly important as certain therapeutic options such as dopamine agonists (DA) have specific contraindications. If the patient is not drug naïve, and has previously consumed dopaminergic medication, it is critical to understand what medications have been tried, at what dose, side effects experienced, and if discontinued, the possible reasons for discontinuation. An understanding of this may help to avoid unnecessary subjection of the patient to therapies that are unlikely to work for them.

Considering that the treatment of PD lasts the entire life span of the patient, thorough counseling is paramount. The patient and caregiver must be explained about the disease, course of the illness, and options for management, i.e., medical, surgical, and additional nonpharmacological approaches such as physiotherapy. Realistic expectations should be set about the extent of improvement with medication, along with the possible side-effect profiles of drugs. The importance of regular follow-up visits and the need for frequent adjustment of treatment regimen must also be explained. Patients should also be encouraged to maintain records of response to medication and report any adverse effects even if relatively minor. In addition, the patient and caregiver should be informed about PD support groups, as this may help them to gain better coping strategies and support. This will also aid in destigmatization and better acceptance of the illness. Availability of disability benefits such as pension, tax-benefits, etc., should also be informed to the patient. Finally, they should be encouraged to participate in research studies and clinical trials.

MEDICAL MANAGEMENT OF MOTOR SYMPTOMS

The *sine qua non* of PD—bradykinesia, rigidity, and rest tremor are certainly observed in early PD, however, they may not be as overt and obvious as in the later stages. These symptoms can be subtle and nonspecific. For instance, patients can complain of clumsiness, dragging of the foot while walking, change in handwriting, mild reduction in arm swing, etc. As stated earlier, treatment strategies often need to be highly individualized and influenced by patient's specific factors. It is imperative to understand that at present treatment options predominantly lead to symptomatic improvement and the medication used for the treatment of early PD is the same as in later stages, albeit in different dosages and combinations.[14] A suggested approach to medical management is provided in **Flowchart 1** and drugs commonly used are listed in **Table 1**.

Levodopa

Replacement of the dopaminergic deficit with levodopa is and will perhaps always persist to be the mainstay and gold standard of pharmacological treatment in PD. Levodopa has consistent and clear evidence of reducing disability and no other drug matched up to the benefits obtained from levodopa.[15-17] Levodopa is typically available as a combination of levodopa and a decarboxylase inhibitor such as carbidopa in order to reduce peripheral conversion and increase central availability of levodopa.

In patients with early PD, levodopa should be considered in the following situations:[18]

- Motor symptoms are significant and interfere with activities of daily living.
- Patients who might be more susceptible to adverse effects of other medications.
- Inability to afford other forms of medication

Treatment should follow a "start slow" and "go slow" regimen, which suggests initiation of a low dose (1/2 tablet of 100/25 or 100/10 levodopa/carbidopa) and slow upward titration based on observed clinical response and occurrence of adverse effects. For better absorption, levodopa should be prescribed either half-hour before or an hour-and-a half after meals. In the event that levodopa produces nausea, light snacks—not rich in protein might be consumed before taking the medication. Domperidone may be additionally prescribed half-hour to prior to levodopa for a few weeks, i.e., until the patient can tolerate levodopa. A levodopa

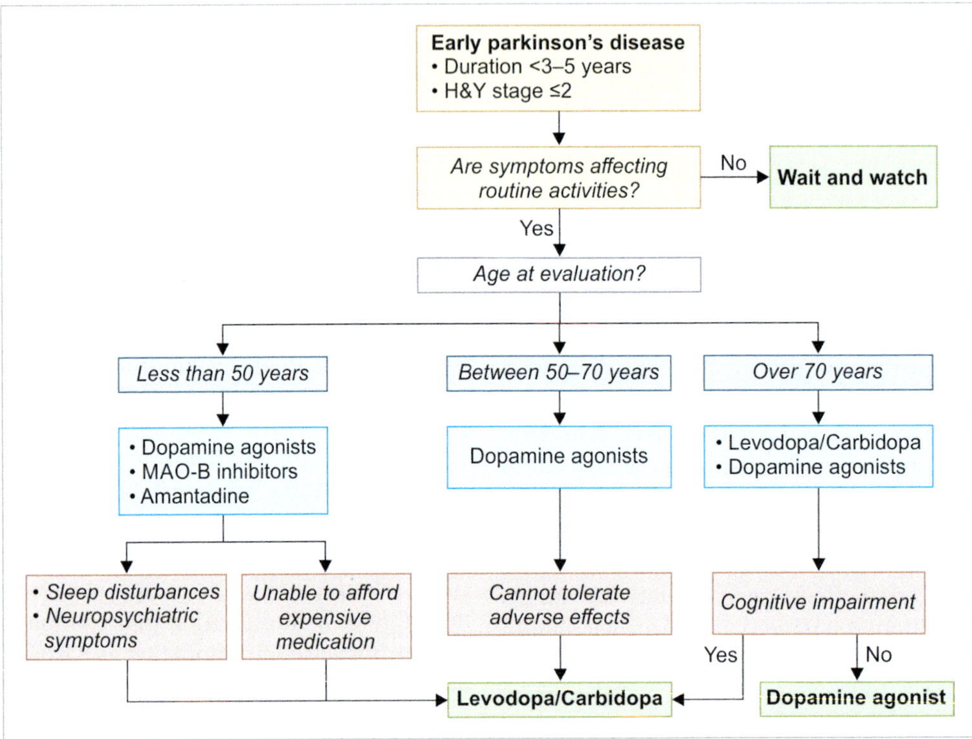

FLOWCHART 1: Treatment approach in early Parkinson's disease.

(H&Y: Hoehn and Yahr)

TABLE 1: Drugs commonly used in the treatment of early Parkinson's disease.

Drug	Starting dose	Maintenance dose	Side effects
Levodopa	½ tablet 100/25 mg or 100/10 mg of levodopa/carbidopa	600 mg/day	Nausea and postural hypotension
Dopamine agonists:			
Pramipexole	0.125 mg TID	0.75–3 mg/day	Daytime somnolence, pedal edema, neuropsychiatric symptoms, impulse control disorders, postural hypotension, and giddiness
Ropinirole	0.25 mg TID	9–24 mg/day	Same as above
Piribedil	50 mg/day	• 150–300 mg/day (monotherapy) • 150 mg/day (adjunct to levodopa)	Same as above
Rotigotine	2 mg/24 hours patch	6 mg/24 hours patch	Same as above

Continued

Continued

Drug	Starting dose	Maintenance dose	Side effects
MAO-B inhibitors:			
Rasagiline	0.5 mg OD	1 mg/day	Worsen dopaminergic adverse effects, increase dyskinesia, confusion, hallucinations, serotonin syndrome
Selegiline	5 mg OD	5–10 mg/day	Same as above
Safinamide	50 mg OD	100 mg/day (OD)	Nausea, insomnia, and hypertension
NMDA receptor blocker:			
Amantadine	100 mg OD	200–400 mg/day	Hallucinations, confusion, nightmares, ankle edema, livedo reticularis, dry mouth, and hyponatremia
Anticholinergics:			
THP	2 mg OD	6 mg/day	Dry mouth, postural giddiness, blurred vision, urinary retention, constipation, and confusion
Benztropine	0.5 mg OD	6 mg/day	Same as above

(COMT: catechol-O-methyl transferase; MAO-B: monoamine oxidase type B; NMDA: N-methyl-D-aspartate; OD: once daily; TID: three times a day; THP: trihexyphenidyl)

daily dose of <600 mg may aid in delaying motor complications,[19,20] which are known to be more common in younger patients with PD.[21] If needed, additional medication such as DAs or monoamine oxidase type B (MAO-B) inhibitors should be considered in lieu of increasing the dose of levodopa.

Continuous dopaminergic stimulation (CDS) is a treatment strategy which aims to mimic the continuous stimulation of dopaminergic receptors seen in normal physiological conditions.[22] The intermittent pulsatile fluctuations produced by dopaminergic medication results in pulsatile stimulation of the receptors, molecular changes in striatal neurons, and physiological changes to pallidal neurons which are thought to contribute to development of motor complications. These alterations have led to the thought that continuous delivery may lead to a reduced risk of motor fluctuations. In this context, the use of controlled release preparations may be theoretically beneficial in patients with early PD.

Dopamine Agonists

Dopamine agonists play a significant role in the management of early PD, particularly due to its utility in levodopa-sparing strategies. They have well-reported efficacy and can be used as monotherapy in early PD. Nonergot DAs, i.e., pramipexole, ropinirole, and rotigotine are primarily used and preferred over ergot DAs such as bromocriptine, lisuride, pergolide, and cabergoline owing to the highest side effect profile of ergot Das.[14,23-25] DAs are preferred in younger patients as it delays the onset of levodopa-induced dyskinesias and more importantly, younger patients can better tolerate DAs.

Dopamine agonists should be at a very-low dose with a slow increase in dose to improve tolerability. For example, pramipexole can be initiated at 0.125 mg TID for a week, following a gradual increase to 0.125 mg per week, till a dose of 0.5 mg TID is achieved. Ropinirole is generally tolerated till a dose of 9–24 mg/day. Rotigotine has the unique benefit of being available as a transdermal patch, providing the option of continuous drug delivery and the probable benefits of CDS. Piribedil is a D2 and D3 agonist which is reported to be well tolerated even in older patients, and can be prescribed as 150–300 mg/day monotherapy or 150 mg/day as adjunct therapy to levodopa.[26]

Despite the seemingly beneficial nature of DAs, the utility is restricted owing to the troublesome adverse effect profile. These include daytime somnolence, pedal edema, neuropsychiatric and cognitive side effects, impulse control disorders, and postural hypotension dizziness.[14,27] In-depth history and clinical assessment should be carried out to rule out psychosis or postural hypotension prior to prescribing DAs. Additionally, they should be used in caution in those with occupations such as drivers, heavy machine operators, etc.

Monoamine Oxidase Type B Inhibitors

Monoamine oxidase type B inhibitors are often used as a first-line therapy for patients with mild motor symptoms. Rasagiline has been proven to be beneficial as monotherapy at 1 mg/day in the TEMPO and LARGO trials, and gained popularity owing to the possibility of a disease-modifying effect leading to the ADAGIO trial.[28-30] However, owing to the lack of long-term benefits of early start rasagiline, this is no longer suggested as a disease-modifying drug. Selegiline has been shown to delay the onset of initiation of levodopa, without any neuroprotective benefits.[6] Although safinamide is primarily used for patients with motor fluctuations, it may be used in early PD as monotherapy at 1 mg/kg/day or in combination with levodopa.[31] In comparison to DAs, MAO-B inhibitors are reported to have a better side-effect profile and may be better tolerated.

Nondopaminergic Agents

N-methyl-D-Aspartate Receptor Blockers

Amantadine is a drug that is commonly used in the late stages of PD for its antidyskinetic effect, however, it can be used as either monotherapy or adjunct therapy in early PD. Patients can be given a dose of 200–400 mg/day divided into two to three doses. If available, extended-release preparations can be administered once a day. Utmost caution should be used in prescribing amantadine to older patients as it has wide side-effect profile including ankle edema, confusion, nightmares, dryness of the mouth, livedo reticularis, and hyponatremia.

Anticholinergics

This group of drugs is particularly useful in young patients with tremor-dominant PD. Trihexyphenidyl at 2 mg OD, increased till 2 mg TID, and benztropine at 0.5 mg OD, increased till 2 mg tid, are known to significantly reduce tremor. However, the utility is limited owing to the lack of benefit on rigidity and bradykinesia. In addition, there are significant and common adverse effects particularly in the elderly which includes dry mouth, dry eyes, psychosis, postural giddiness, psychosis, cognitive impairment, urinary hesitancy and constipation.[14] Despite the utility of anticholinergics in reducing tremor, they should not be prescribed as first-line drugs or used as monotherapy. Apart from the tremor reducing potential, these drugs may be helpful in patients with associated dystonia.

Medications under Evaluation for Use in Early Parkinson's Disease

In early PD, response to medication is satisfactory with the above list of well-established medications. However, efforts are persistently made to find drugs to optimize treatment. A few ongoing studies[32] include the evaluation of:

- *Tavapadon:* A novel D1/D5 dopamine receptor partial agonist—phase 3 studies to evaluate the effect on motor functions in early and late PD.
- *P2B001:* It is a combination of low-dose pramipexole and rasagiline. Phase 2 trials show good clinical efficacy with no increase in adverse effects.
- *Opicapone:* A well-established catechol-O-methyltransferase inhibitor frequently used in patients with motor fluctuations, it is currently being evaluated to assess benefits in patients with early PD.

MEDICAL MANAGEMENT OF NON-MOTOR SYMPTOMS

Non-motor symptoms form a significant component of the overall symptomatology of early PD, with several NMS preceding the onset of motor symptoms, i.e., premotor symptoms of hyposmia, REM (rapid eye movement) behavior disorder (RBD), and constipation. Although they are certainly more pronounced and severe in late or advanced PD, even in early PD, they significantly impact the overall quality of life. Patients with early PD may often present with a range of NMS. This can include olfactory dysfunction in the form of hyposmia, sleep symptoms which include RBD and excessive daytime sleepiness, neuropsychiatric symptoms such as depression and anxiety, and other NMS such as fatigue, pain, and sensory symptoms. Comprehensive management of the patient requires awareness of NMS in addition to motor symptoms.

Medications used for the management of motor symptoms may often have beneficial effects on NMS, leading to a reduction in the need for polypharmacy.[32] For example, safinamide has been shown to improve sleep, fatigue, mood, and pain.[33] It is imperative to understand that several practical approaches routinely followed in clinical practice may not appear to be recommended practices from an evidence-based medicine perspective and there are no standardized guidelines for recommended dosage in PD.[34] This may be attributable to lack of studies evaluating the effect of these medications in patients with PD.

Neuropsychiatric Symptoms

No specific guidelines exist for management of depression; however, selective serotonin reuptake inhibitors and selective norepinephrine reuptake inhibitors are useful and frequently used **(Table 2)**. Tricyclic antidepressants are infrequently used in older patients due to higher adverse effects such as orthostatic hypotension, constipation, confusion, and occasionally delirium.[15]

Current trials include the evaluation of vortioxetine (a serotonin receptor and transport modulator), psilocybin, intravenous ketamine, and the comparison of nortriptyline and escitalopram in the treatment of depression in PD.[32]

Sleep Symptoms

Clonazepam is the drug of choice for treatment of RBD in PD. However, melatonin may be used in patients who cannot tolerate or have contradictions to clonazepam.[35] For patients with PD and excessive daytime sleepiness, modafinil is the mainstay of treatment.[36]

TABLE 2: Pharmacological treatment of nonmotor symptoms in early Parkinson's disease (PD).

Medication	Starting dose	Maximum dose	Remarks
Neuropsychiatric symptoms			
Depression:			
Selective serotonin reuptake inhibitors:			
Sertraline	25 mg HS	100 mg/day	Hyponatremia
Escitalopram	5 mg/day	20 mg/day	Avoid prescribing with MAO-B inhibitors
Selective norepinephrine reuptake inhibitors:			
Duloxetine	20 mg/day	60 mg/day	• Constipation • Avoid prescribing with MAO-B inhibitors
Impulse control disorders: Gradually taper and stop dopamine agonists			
Sleep symptoms			
REM sleep behavior disorder:			
Clonazepam	0.25 mg HS	0.5–1 mg HS	Excessive daytime drowsiness
Melatonin	3 mg HS	6–15 mg HS	• Excessive daytime drowsiness • Altered circadian rhythm
Excessive daytime sleepiness:			
Modafinil	100 mg/day (morning)	200 mg/day (morning)	-
Gastrointestinal symptoms			
Constipation: High fiber diet, lactulose, sodium-picosulfate, or polyethylene glycol			
Other symptoms			
Pain: Optimization of dopaminergic therapy			

(HS: at bedtime; MAO-B: monoamine oxidase type B)

Gastrointestinal Symptoms

Although constipation is a known premotor symptom in PD, it may often be secondary to treatment with anticholinergic medication. In which case, the anticholinergic drugs should be stopped. Lactulose, sodium-picosulfate, or polyethylene glycol may be used to alleviate constipation. Additionally, domperidone, tegaserod, and mosapride are useful prokinetic agents.[37] Recently, ENT-1, an oral compound inhibiting formation of α-synuclein aggregates, has been shown to reduce constipation in addition to improving cognitive and psychosis-related outcomes.[38] Other substances under evaluation include pyridostigmine and probiotics.[32]

Other Symptoms

Pain is most often related to multiple factors such as rigidity and akinesia, hence, responds frequently to optimization of dopaminergic treatment.[37] Due to the involvement of the dopaminergic system in the pain observed in PD, oral opicapone, and subcutaneous apomorphine are under evaluation for treatment of pain in PD.[32]

DISEASE-MODIFYING THERAPIES

Although the symptomatic treatment of PD has grown over the years, the core group of drugs will invariability remain the same. Disease-modifying therapies which aim to modulate disease progression by targeting the fundamental root of the disease will eventually modify the treatment landscape. Discussing current trials is beyond the scope of this chapter, however, it is beneficial to be aware of current approaches and targets for disease-modifying therapy. Some approaches for disease modification include:[32,39]

- Targeting specific proteins (LRRK2 and GCase) or organelles (mitochondria and lysosomes)
- *Reduction of α-synuclein*: Influencing production, turnover, aggregation, and propagation.
- Influence downstream mechanisms—neuronal survival or immunomodulation.

These are of particular importance owing to the growing relevance of genetic subtypes of PD. For instance, targeting *LRRK2*, or mitochondria which is related to *Parkin* and *PINK1*, or glucocerebrosidase (*GBA*) gene therapies.[32]

MONITORING PATIENTS ON TREATMENT

As mentioned earlier, patients with early PD require regular follow-up and close monitoring of response to treatment along with evaluation of progression of symptoms particularly the emergence of red flag signs which could be indicative of atypical parkinsonism **(Box 3)**. Although regular in-person assessment of motor symptoms is crucial, telemedicine may be an appropriate adjunct to permit more frequent reporting of treatment response, NMS, and any medication related adverse effects.

BOX 3: Red flags suggesting a parkinsonian disorder other than Parkinson's disease.

- Vertical gaze impairment
- Nuchal dystonia
- Early impairment of postural reflexes—falls
- Significant abnormalities of gait—freezing
- Disturbances in ocular motility—vertical gaze palsy
- Autonomic dysfunction unrelated to drugs
- Progressive cognitive impairment
- Neuropsychiatric symptoms—psychosis
- Cerebellar signs
- Unresponsiveness to levodopa

Patients may often be curious about deep brain stimulation (DBS) as a treatment option. It is essential to explain the stage of illness and situation where DBS is usually considered, which is typically in advanced stages of PD in association with motor fluctuations and dyskinesias. However, there are specific situations such as patients with severe tremor dominant PD or those who develop levodopa induced dyskinesias even with very low doses of levodopa where DBS may be considered even in the early stages.[40]

CONCLUSION

The treatment of early PD is challenging and requires keen attention to be paid to numerous factors beyond the motor symptoms that a patient presents with. Therapeutic benefit has to be balanced again NMS, side-effect profiles, and socioeconomic considerations. Developing a good rapport with the patient and setting realistic expectations is crucial to ensure compliance to treatment. The therapeutic landscape of PD is steadily changing and is perhaps likely to see drastic changes in the future with the advent of reliable disease-modifying therapies.

REFERENCES

1. Adwani S, Yadav R, Kumar K, Chandra SR, Pal PK. Neuropsychological profile in early Parkinson's disease: Comparison between patients with right side onset versus left side onset of motor symptoms. Ann Indian Acad Neurol. 2016;19(1):74-8.
2. Ascherio A, Schwarzschild MA. The epidemiology of Parkinson's disease: risk factors and prevention. Lancet Neurol. 2016;15(12):1257-72.
3. Szewczyk-Krolikowski K, Tomlinson P, Nithi K, Wade-Martins R, Talbot K, Ben-Shlomo Y, et al. The influence of age and gender on motor and non-motor features of early Parkinson's disease: initial findings from the Oxford Parkinson Disease Center (OPDC) discovery cohort. Parkinsonism Relat Disord. 2014;20(1):99-105.
4. Reimão S, Pita Lobo P, Neutel D, Correia Guedes L, Coelho M, et al. Substantia nigra neuromelanin magnetic resonance imaging in de novo Parkinson's disease patients. Eur J Neurol. 2015;22(3):540-6.
5. Kang JH, Mollenhauer B, Coffey CS, Toledo JB, Weintraub D, Galasko DR, et al. CSF biomarkers associated with disease heterogeneity in early Parkinson's disease: the Parkinson's Progression Markers Initiative study. Acta Neuropathol. 2016;131(6):935-49.
6. Steering D. DATATOP: a multicenter controlled clinical trial in early Parkinson's disease. Arch Neurol. 1989;46(10):1052-60.
7. Hristova AH, Koller WC. Early Parkinson's disease: what is the best approach to treatment. Drugs Aging. 2000;17(3):165-81.
8. Postuma RB, Berg D, Stern M, Poewe W, Olanow CW, Oertel W, et al. MDS clinical diagnostic criteria for Parkinson's disease. Mov Disord. 2015;30(12):1591-601.
9. de Bie RM, Clarke CE, Espay AJ, Fox SH, Lang AE. Initiation of pharmacological therapy in Parkinson's disease: when, why, and how. Lancet Neurol. 2020;19(5):452-61.
10. Aminoff MJ. Treatment should not be initiated too soon in Parkinson's disease. Ann Neurol. 2006;59(3):562-4.
11. Schapira AH, Obeso J. Timing of treatment initiation in Parkinson's disease: a need for reappraisal? Ann Neurol. 2006;59(3):559-62.
12. Löhle M, Ramberg CJ, Reichmann H, Schapira AH. Early versus delayed initiation of pharmacotherapy in Parkinson's disease. Drugs. 2014;74:645-57.
13. Stocchi F, Vacca L, Radicati FG. How to optimize the treatment of early stage Parkinson's disease. Transl Neurodegener. 2015;4:4.
14. Sy MAC, Fernandez HH. Pharmacological treatment of early motor manifestations of Parkinson disease (PD). Neurotherapeutics. 2020;17(4):1331-8.
15. Connolly BS, Lang AE. Pharmacological treatment of Parkinson disease: a review. JAMA. 2014;311(16):1670-83.
16. Ferreira JJ, Katzenschlager R, Bloem BR, Bonuccelli U, Burn D, Deuschl G, et al. Summary of the recommendations of the EFNS/MDS-ES review on therapeutic management of Parkinson's disease. Eur J Neurol. 2013;20(1):5-15.
17. Poewe W, Antonini A, Zijlmans JC, Burkhard PR, Vingerhoets F. Levodopa in the treatment of Parkinson's disease: an old drug still going strong. Clin interve aging. 2010;5:229-38.
18. Pahwa R, Lyons KE. Treatment of early Parkinson's disease. Curr Opin Neurol. 2014;27(4):442-9.
19. Hauser RA, Auinger P, Oakes D, Parkinson Study G. Levodopa response in early Parkinson's disease. Mov Disord. 2009;24(16):2328-36.
20. Group PS. Levodopa and the progression of Parkinson's disease. N Engl J Med. 2004;2004(351): 2498-508.
21. Wickremaratchi MM, Ben-Shlomo Y, Morris HR. The effect of onset age on the clinical features of Parkinson's disease. Eur J Neurol. 2009;16(4): 450-6.
22. Olanow CW, Calabresi P, Obeso JA. Continuous dopaminergic stimulation as a treatment for Parkinson's disease: current status and future opportunities. Movement Disord. 2020;35(10): 1731-44.
23. Kieburtz K, Parkinson Study Group Prami BIDI. Twice-daily, low-dose pramipexole in early Parkinson's disease: a randomized, placebo-controlled trial. Mov Disord. 2011;26(1):37-44.
24. Hauser RA, Schapira AH, Rascol O, Barone P, Mizuno Y, Salin L, et al. Randomized, double-blind, multicenter evaluation of pramipexole extended release once daily in early Parkinson's disease. Mov Disord. 2010;25(15):2542-9.
25. Adler CH, Sethi KD, Hauser RA, Davis TL, Hammerstad JP, Bertoni J, et al. Ropinirole for the treatment of early Parkinson's disease. The Ropinirole Study Group. Neurology. 1997;49(2): 393-9.

26. Rascol O, Dubois B, Caldas AC, Senn S, Del Signore S, Lees A. Early piribedil monotherapy of Parkinson's disease: A planned seven-month report of the REGAIN study. Mov disord. 2006;21(12):2110-5.
27. Antonini A, Tolosa E, Mizuno Y, Yamamoto M, Poewe WH. A reassessment of risks and benefits of dopamine agonists in Parkinson's disease. Lancet Neurol. 2009;8(10):929-37.
28. Viallet F, Pitel S, Lancrenon S, Blin O. Evaluation of the safety and tolerability of rasagiline in the treatment of the early stages of Parkinson's disease. Curr med res opin. 2013;29(1):23-31.
29. Olanow CW, Rascol O, Hauser R, Feigin PD, Jankovic J, Lang A, et al. A double-blind, delayed-start trial of rasagiline in Parkinson's disease. N Engl J Med. 2009;361(13):1268-78.
30. Rascol O, Fitzer-Attas CJ, Hauser R, Jankovic J, Lang A, Langston JW, et al. A double-blind, delayed-start trial of rasagiline in Parkinson's disease (the ADAGIO study): prespecified and post-hoc analyses of the need for additional therapies, changes in UPDRS scores, and non-motor outcomes. Lancet Neurol. 2011;10(5):415-23.
31. Bette S, Shpiner DS, Singer C, Moore H. Safinamide in the management of patients with Parkinson's disease not stabilized on levodopa: a review of the current clinical evidence. Ther clin risk manag. 2018;14:1737-45.
32. Wolff A, Schumacher NU, Pürner D, Machetanz G, Demleitner AF, Feneberg E, et al. Parkinson's disease therapy: what lies ahead? J Neural Trans (Vienna). 2023;130(6):793-820.
33. Stocchi F, Antonini A, Berg D, Bergmans B, Jost WH, Katzenschlager R, et al. Safinamide in the treatment pathway of Parkinson's disease: a European Delphi consensus. npj Parkinson's Disease. 2022;8(1):17.
34. Van Wamelen DJ, Rukavina K, Podlewska AM, Chaudhuri KR. Advances in the pharmacological and non-pharmacological management of non-motor symptoms in Parkinson's disease: an update since 2017. Curr Neuropharmacol. 2023;21(8):1786-805.
35. Aurora RN, Zak RS, Maganti RK, Auerbach SH, Casey KR, Chowdhuri S, et al. Best practice guide for the treatment of REM sleep behavior disorder (RBD). J Clin Sleep Med. 2010;6(1):85-95.
36. Zesiewicz TA, Sullivan KL, Arnulf I, Chaudhuri KR, Morgan JC, Gronseth GS, et al. Practice Parameter: treatment of nonmotor symptoms of Parkinson disease: report of the Quality Standards Subcommittee of the American Academy of Neurology. Neurology. 2010;74(11):924-31.
37. Sprenger F, Poewe W. Management of motor and non-motor symptoms in Parkinson's disease. CNS Drugs. 2013;27(4):259-72.
38. Camilleri M, Subramanian T, Pagan F, Isaacson S, Gil R, Hauser RA, et al. Oral ENT-01 targets enteric neurons to treat constipation in Parkinson disease: a randomized controlled trial. Ann intern med. 2022;175(12):1666-74.
39. Vijiaratnam N, Simuni T, Bandmann O, Morris HR, Foltynie T. Progress towards therapies for disease modification in Parkinson's disease. Lancet Neurol. 2021;20(7):559-72.
40. Hartmann CJ, Fliegen S, Groiss SJ, Wojtecki L, Schnitzler A. An update on best practice of deep brain stimulation in Parkinson's disease. Ther Adv Neurol Disord. 2019;12:1756286419838096.

CHAPTER 2

Current Medical Management of Advanced Parkinson's Disease

Karthik Harisankar, Sahil Mehta

ABSTRACT

Advanced Parkinson's disease is defined by the presence of motor complications as well as non-motor features of dementia, psychosis, and dysautonomia. Significant progress has been made in Parkinson's disease in the last decade, leading to the discovery of novel agents to treat motor fluctuations and dyskinesias by targeting dopaminergic and nondopaminergic pathways. Novel modes of delivery bypassing problems of gastrointestinal absorption, such as inhalational, subcutaneous, and even buccal mucosa, are being utilized to tackle the motor and non-motor complications which contribute to significant disability in advanced Parkinson's disease (PD).

Keywords: Advanced Parkinson's disease, Motor complications, Fluctuations, Dyskinesias, Autonomic dysfunction, Psychosis, Freezing of gait.

INTRODUCTION

Advanced Parkinson's disease (PD) was previously defined as Hoen and Yahr stage 4 or 5.[1] This clinical definition has certain limitations, as it does not consider the contribution of non-motor symptoms and the quality of life impacted by the disease. Recently, Delphi criteria have been introduced based on the OBSERVE-PD (OBSERVational, cross-sEctional PD) study, which includes 11 criteria, including levodopa dosing, sleep disturbances, falls, dementia, and psychosis, apart from motor fluctuations.[2] Advanced PD encompasses at least one of the following:[3]

- Dependence for activities of daily living despite optimum levodopa therapy
- Significant postural instability with a tendency to or presence of falls
- Freezing of gait
- Pronounced postural deformity
- The presence of motor and nonmotor complications (fluctuations, dyskinesias, dementia, and psychosis)

The most characteristic feature of advanced PD is motor complications. A combination of disease progression and fluctuating levodopa levels are primarily responsible for the motor complications of PD.[4] Once they occur, motor complications are usually irreversible. They can be categorized as fluctuations and dyskinesias **(Table 1)**.

Although the exact reason for fluctuations is not apparent, different mechanisms are proposed:[5]

- Decrease in dopamine storage capacity as the disease reaches advanced stages.
- Alterations in postsynaptic dopamine receptors by free radicals which lead to irreversible changes.

TABLE 1: Motor fluctuations.

Fluctuation	Explanation
Early "wearing-off"	Defined to be present when an adequate dosage of levodopa does not last at least 4 hours
Sudden "off"/Random "off"	Parkinsonism develops over minutes rather than 10s of minutes, and they are less predictable in terms of timing with the dosing of levodopa
Delayed "on"	Levodopa takes longer than 30 minutes after being swallowing for it to have effect
Episodic failure to respond (dose failure)	Failure of the patient to respond to a dose of levodopa; no-on
Response varies in relationship to meals	Levodopa concentrations in plasma are delayed when the medication is taken in the fed state
Weak response at end of the day	Diurnal variation in their responsiveness to levodopa. Often, the patient reports that she or he does the best after the first morning dose, and the response is less as the day wears on

- Standard levodopa treatment leads to pulsatile and nonphysiological dopamine concentrations in the striatum.

DYSKINESIAS

Levodopa-induced dyskinesia (LID) is classified as peak-dose dyskinesia, wearing-off or off-period dyskinesia, and diphasic dyskinesia.[5] The most common phenomenon is chorea. Rarely, it takes the form of ballism. More commonly, patients present with a combination of chorea and dystonia. The following reasons are attributed to dyskinesias:[6]

- Nigrostriatal degeneration and pulsatile dopaminergic stimulation
- Altered dopamine receptor-mediated signaling
- Maladaptive plasticity
- Abnormal glutamatergic and serotoninergic neurotransmission

Treatment of Motor Fluctuations Associated with Levodopa Therapy

A good history and examination to elicit the exact type of motor complication are essential, so the clinician can identify and provide effective treatment suggestions. This requires the participation of both the patient and the caregiver. Substituting levodopa with dopamine agonists can diminish the severity of motor complications. However, this does not eliminate them and occurs at the cost of worsening Parkinsonism.

Wearing-off

The onset of wearing-off can be delayed by using dopamine agonists and postponing the introduction of levodopa.[7] Monoamine oxidase-B (MAO-B) inhibitors like selegiline and rasagiline potentiate the action of levodopa.[8] Selegiline is introduced at 5 mg once daily and increased to 5 mg twice daily, as necessary. Side effects include confusion and psychosis, particularly in older people and dyskinesias. Rasagiline decreases the daily "off" time by about 1 hour daily.[9] Safinamide, apart from being a reversible MAO-B inhibitor, also blocks sodium channels and modulates glutamate release. It has been shown to improve off periods in a dose of 100 mg/day without increasing troublesome dyskinesias and was approved by the Food and Drug Administration (FDA) in 2017.[10]

A controlled-release (CR) preparation of levodopa can also be effective in patients with mild wearing-off.[11] Patients can gradually switch from standard carbidopa/levodopa to CR. However, during this switch, the following things need to be considered.

- Controlled release preparation of levodopa takes about an hour to become effective, so most patients require additional immediate release of levodopa to get an optimal response.
- Due to the variability in absorption and bioavailability, 100 mg of levodopa in standard immediate release of levodopa/carbidopa is equivalent to 130–150 mg of levodopa CR.

The controlled release preparation is generally used in treating nocturnal akinesia, and early-morning offs in advanced-stage PD patients. Another strategy is to give standard carbidopa/levodopa at more frequent intervals.

Catechol-O-methyltransferase (COMT) inhibitors increase the "on" time by about an hour daily. Entacapone, available as a 200 mg tablet, is given simultaneously with each dose of carbidopa/levodopa.[12] Entacapone can cause urine discoloration, which patients should know before starting. Other COMT inhibitors like tolcapone are rarely used given their unacceptable side effects, which include hepatitis and explosive diarrhea. A novel once-daily third-generation COMT inhibitor, opicapone, received FDA approval in April 2020 for motor fluctuations based on BIPARK-I and II randomized clinical trials.[13,14] A dose of 50 mg reduced the mean-off time by 50 minutes, with the benefits maintained for up to 1 year in open-label extension studies. Adverse effects include dyskinesias, insomnia, and elevated creatine phosphokinase levels.

Istradefylline is an adenosine A2A receptor antagonist. It is approved by the FDA to treat off periods in advanced PD as an adjunct to levodopa/carbidopa. Istradefylline blocks adenosine A2A receptors in the brain, enhancing dopamine D2 receptor-mediated neurotransmission. Randomized, double-blind, and placebo-controlled studies have shown that this drug significantly reduced "off" time by approximately 1 hour/day compared to placebo.[15] Patients reported improved motor function during "on" time without troublesome dyskinesia. It is available in 20- or 40-mg doses. The most common adverse effect of istradefylline is dyskinesia.

The addition of all these therapies carries the risk of developing dyskinesias; in that case, the dosage of carbidopa/levodopa needs to be reduced. The FDA approved the extended-release of levodopa-carbidopa formulation (Rytary) in 2015 based on three phase III double-blind randomized clinical trials.[16] It contains both immediate-release and extended-release beads of carbidopa/levodopa that are released at different rates. Compared with immediate release of levodopa, it reduces daily off time without increasing troublesome dyskinesia.

Sudden "Offs"/Random "Offs"

Subcutaneous injections of the dopamine agonist apomorphine are effective in treating sudden-offs.[17] Its onset of action is around 5 minutes and lasts for an hour. Domperidone is taken before the injection to prevent nausea and vomiting. Another strategy is to dissolve levodopa in carbonated water and drink it, which shows its effect in about 10–15 minutes.

Inhaled levodopa (Inbrija) was approved in 2018 to treat off periods. It reaches peak plasma concentration at 5 minutes, bypassing the slow gastrointestinal absorption of oral levodopa. It effectively reduces off periods and improves UPDRS III scores by a mean of 3.9 points compared to placebo.[18,19] A dose of 84 mg of levodopa (two capsules of 42 mg each) is administered via a breath-actuated inhaler. The maximum approved doses per day is 5. Adverse effects include dry cough, and this drug is contraindicated in patients with asthma or chronic obstructive airway disease.

Dose Failures

This occurs primarily due to poor gastric emptying and can be overcome using liquid levodopa preparations. Another approach is to use apomorphine injections.[20]

Delayed On

This is usually encountered with the first dose in the morning and occurs due to the low affinity of dopamine receptors. It can be treated by dissolving levodopa before ingesting to obtain higher levodopa concentrations in the plasma sooner.

Weak Response at the End of the Day

This can be combated by increasing the afternoon and evening doses of levodopa. A controlled-release preparation of levodopa, a dopamine agonist, anticholinergics, or amantadine can also be added to the existing regimen.

Response Varies in Relation to Meals

It is well known that levodopa has to be spaced for at least 45 minutes to 1 hour with the meals due to the problem of delayed gastric emptying in PD. In rare patients, high-protein meals interfere with the response to levodopa. This can be tackled by skipping protein-rich meals for breakfast and lunch and taking high-protein quantities at dinner time.[21]

Treatment of Dyskinesias

Peak-dose Dyskinesias

This problem can be resolved by reducing the individual dose with more frequent intervals to counteract the reduced benefit of lowering the dose alone. Another method is to substitute higher doses of a dopamine agonist while decreasing the dose of levodopa. Dopamine agonists have a lower propensity to cause dyskinesias than levodopa.

Continuous release of levodopa can also be tried in patients by lowering the peak plasma levels of levodopa. However, the slow decay in plasma levels can cause long-lasting dyskinesias.

If these strategies do not work, amantadine can be tried. It has anti-glutaminergic effects and a dose-dependent anti-dyskinetic effect.[22] Amantadine can be started at 100 mg twice a day and increased gradually up to 200 mg twice a day as needed.

Another drug that can be used is "Clozapine." It is an atypical antipsychotic that does not worsen "Parkinsonism." Clozapine has been shown to alleviate levodopa-induced dyskinesias and increase "on" time.[23] The baseline absolute neutrophil count (ANC) should be 1,500/mm^3 before starting the drug. Regular ANC monitoring (Weekly for 6 months, biweekly for 6 months, followed by monthly) is needed. Start with 12.5 mg once or twice daily and titrate slowly with divided doses.

Side effects of clozapine include:

- Orthostatic hypotension
- Bradycardia
- Syncope
- Seizures
- Myocarditis and cardiomyopathy
- Anticholinergic side effects

DIPHASIC DYSKINESIA

Diphasic dyskinesia develops at the rise and fall of plasma levodopa levels. Typically seen to involve the legs, this phenomenon is complex to explain. The most effective approach is to utilize a longer-acting dopamine agonist as the primary therapeutic agent and levodopa as the supplementary drug. Levodopa/carbidopa intestinal gel (LCIG) may also be helpful in such a scenario. There is robust evidence to show that LCIG decreases off time and increases on time without dyskinesia.[24]

Off-dystonia

It typically occurs in the early morning before the first dose of the drug and usually involves the leg. Usually, a long-acting formulation of levodopa at bedtime suffices.

Combination of Fluctuations and Dyskinesias (Yo-yo-ing)

Medications with a longer half-life than levodopa are preferred to smooth out the motor fluctuations. Dopamine agonists are employed as the primary therapeutic agent with judicious use of carbidopa/levodopa. Intraduodenal levodopa pump therapy and apomorphine infusions can also be helpful. Deep brain stimulation surgery remains an option in such cases of fluctuations.

Treatment of Autonomic Dysfunction in Advanced Parkinson's Disease

Autonomic dysfunction in patients with PD can cause urogenital dysfunction and affect blood pressure, the gastrointestinal tract, and the skin.

Urogenital Dysfunction

The most common complaint is increased urine frequency, especially at night, and urgency.[25] Antimuscarinic drugs such as oxybutynin 5–10 mg at night or 5 mg thrice daily can be helpful if there is no significant post-void residual urine. Reduction of fluid intake at night can decrease nocturia. Tolterodine is another alternative. Tricyclic antidepressants such as amitriptyline, owing to their anticholinergic action, can also be used. β-3-adrenergic receptor antagonist mirabegron produces relaxation of the detrusor muscle.[26] Sildenafil is helpful in the treatment of erectile dysfunction in PD.

Orthostatic Hypotension

The first step in patients with orthostatic hypotension is to increase fluid (3–3.5 L/day) and salt intake (2–3 g/day). Other nonpharmacological approaches include raising the head end at night to prevent supine hypertension and the use of compression stockings or abdominal binders. Fludrocortisone (0.1–0.5 mg) or midodrine (a selective α-agonist) (2.5–5 mg three times a day) can be used to increase blood pressure.[27] Levodopa and dopamine agonists exacerbate postural hypotension, and doses of these need to be optimized. Newer drugs include droxidopa, a prodrug of norepinephrine with a starting dose of 100 mg thrice daily.

Constipation is prevalent in PD, occurring in >80% of cases. It is facilitated by adequate fluid intake, a high-fiber diet, green leafy vegetables, fruits, and lactulose (10–20 g/day) or other mild laxatives. Patients should be advised to stop anticholinergic drugs and increase physical activity. Polyethylene glycol powder can effectively overcome constipation and is given in a dose of 17 g/day dissolved in a glass of water at bedtime.[28] Pyridostigmine can also aid peristalsis by enhancing parasympathetic tone and help to treat constipation.

Drooling saliva can be decreased using peripherally acting anticholinergic drugs such as glycopyrrolate and propantheline. Intraparotid botulinum toxin A injections can sometimes effectively reduce salivary secretions and drooling.[29] Nonpharmacological measures include chewing gum, which also helps with dry mouth.

Cognitive and Psychiatric Manifestations

Dementia and psychosis are common in advanced PD and contribute significantly to morbidity and mortality. Anticholinergic drugs can precipitate cognitive decline and confusion. Withdrawal of such agents is of utmost importance. Donepezil can provide a modest benefit in cognitive functions without worsening motor symptoms. Rivastigmine has shown moderate improvement in dementia associated with PD in large randomized trials. It has the best evidence of efficacy in PD.[30] Memantine can also be used.

Patients with PD tend to have a personality change. Passivity, dependency, and lack of motivation are often seen. It is difficult but essential to make a distinction between apathy and depression. Depression in PD can be treated with selective serotonin reuptake inhibitors (SSRIs). Tricyclic antidepressants like amitriptyline can also be used, although their sedative and anticholinergic potential may precipitate delirium and confusion in elderly patients. Electroconvulsive therapy (ECT) can be used in treatment-resistant depression and has also been shown to improve motor symptoms of PD.[31]

Sometimes, the cause of anxiety in PD is due to the impact of the disease and Parkinsonian symptoms and its effect on life situations. Off-state anxiety is treated by optimizing antiparkinsonian drugs. Persistent symptoms can be treated with SSRIs or buspirone. Anxiety and stress worsen tremors, and a short-acting benzodiazepine can provide relief.

PSYCHOSIS IN PARKINSON'S DISEASE

Psychosis in PD is a result of complex interplay between the progressive pathology affecting the cortical and subcortical pathways, the adverse effects of drugs, and intercurrent infections or metabolic disturbances. The most likely cause in such a scenario is antiparkinsonian drug therapy. Searching for some intercurrent illness, urinary or respiratory tract infection, or other metabolic disturbances is also prudent.

Psychosis as a result of antiparkinsonian medications can usually be managed by gradually withdrawing them in the following order: anticholinergics, amantadine, and MAO-B inhibitors. The dose of dopamine agonists should be reduced or entirely stopped. If the symptoms persist, the dose of levodopa should be tapered at the last.

Atypical antipsychotics, such as quetiapine and clozapine, do not aggravate parkinsonism and can be added in cases of severe psychosis. Quetiapine is used more often due to its safety profile. However, it is effective only for mild-to-moderate psychosis in a starting dose of 25–50 mg at night with a maximum dose of 200–300 mg/day in liaison with the psychiatrist. Clozapine remains another option. It is underutilized because of the need for blood count monitoring. In practice, it has a faster symptomatic benefit. It is started at a dose of 6.25 mg/day dose and increased weekly to a maximum dose of 50 mg/day.

Pimavanserin is a potent 5-HT2A receptor antagonist/inverse agonist and is considered a first-line therapy for managing PD psychosis now.[32,33] However, it is still unavailable in India.

FREEZING OF GAIT

Managing freezing of gait (FOG) requires a multifaceted approach that includes pharmacological, nonpharmacological, and sometimes surgical interventions. FOG occurs more commonly in the off period; thus, optimizing dopaminergic therapies is the first step in its treatment.[34]

This approach is ineffective for gait freezing, which occurs even in the on state. 24-hours levodopa-carbidopa intestinal gel therapy has also been shown to reduce levodopa unresponsive FOG and associated falls.[35]

Physical rehabilitation is crucial, and several approaches can be used. These include action observation training, treadmill training, curved walking training, and supervised slackline training. Behavioral strategies, such as cueing, have been shown to modulate FOG, incorporating visual, auditory, and somatosensory cues and virtual reality in its treatment. The utility of artificial intelligence and wearable technology in managing this difficult-to-treat symptom cannot be overemphasized.[36]

CONCLUSION

In the last decade, newer drugs, formulations, and novel delivery modes have been developed for the management of motor fluctuations and dyskinesias, adding to the therapeutic arsenal of Parkinson's disease. These pharmacological approaches target both dopaminergic and nondopaminergic pathways. However, long-term data is needed to confirm the long-term effectiveness, compliance, and safety profile of these novel agents or modes of administration.

REFERENCES

1. Hoehn MM, Yahr MD. Parkinsonism: onset, progression and mortality. Neurology. 1967;17(5): 427-42.
2. Fasano A, Fung VSC, Lopiano L, Elibol B, Smolentseva IG, Seppi K, et al. Characterizing advanced Parkinson's disease: OBSERVE-PD observational study results of 2615 patients. BMC Neurol. 2019;19(1):50.
3. Jankovic J, Hallett M, Okun MS, Comella CL, Fahn S. Medical management of Parkinson's disease. In: Jankovic J, Hallett M, Okun MS, Comella CL, Fahn S (eds). Principles and Practice of Movement Disorders, 3rd edition. Philadelphia: Elsevier; 2021.
4. Freitas ME, Hess CW, Fox SH. Motor Complications of Dopaminergic Medications in Parkinson's Disease. Semin Neurol. 2017;37(2):147-57.
5. Pandey S, Srivanitchapoom P. Levodopa-induced Dyskinesia: Clinical Features, Pathophysiology, and Medical Management. Ann Indian Acad Neurol. 2017;20(3):190-8.
6. Calabresi P, Di Filippo M, Ghiglieri V, Tambasco N, Picconi B. Levodopa-induced dyskinesias in patients with Parkinson's disease: filling the bench-to-bedside gap. Lancet Neurol. 2010;9(11):1106-17.
7. Woitalla D, Buhmann C, Hilker-Roggendorf R, Höglinger G, Koschel J, Müller T, et al. Role of dopamine agonists in Parkinson's disease therapy. J Neural Transm (Vienna). 2023;130(6):863-73. Erratum in: J Neural Transm (Vienna). 2023.
8. Alborghetti M, Nicoletti F. Different Generations of Type-B Monoamine Oxidase Inhibitors in Parkinson's Disease: From Bench to Bedside. Curr Neuropharmacol. 2019;17(9):861-73.
9. Parkinson Study Group. A randomized placebo-controlled trial of rasagiline in levodopa-treated patients with Parkinson disease and motor fluctuations: the PRESTO study. Arch Neurol. 2005;62(2):241-8.
10. Abbruzzese G, Barone P, Lopiano L, Stocchi F. The Current Evidence for the Use of Safinamide for the Treatment of Parkinson's Disease. Drug Des Devel Ther. 2021;15:2507-17.
11. Koller WC, Pahwa R. Treating motor fluctuations with controlled-release levodopa preparations. Neurology. 1994;44(7 Suppl 6):S23-8.
12. Poewe W. Catechol-O-methyltransferase inhibition with entacapone: Evidence from controlled clinical trials in Parkinson's disease. Eur J Neurol. 2023;30 Suppl 2:9-14.
13. Ferreira JJ, Lees A, Rocha JF, Poewe W, Rascol O, Soares-da-Silva P; Bi-Park 1 investigators. Opicapone as an adjunct to levodopa in patients with Parkinson's disease and end-of-dose motor fluctuations: a randomised, double-blind, controlled trial. Lancet Neurol. 2016;15(2):154-65.
14. Lees AJ, Ferreira J, Rascol O, Poewe W, Rocha JF, McCrory M, et al.; BIPARK-2 Study Investigators. Opicapone as Adjunct to Levodopa Therapy in Patients With Parkinson Disease and Motor Fluctuations: A Randomized Clinical Trial. JAMA Neurol. 2017;74(2):197-206.
15. Jenner P, Mori A, Aradi SD, Hauser RA. Istradefylline—a first generation adenosine A2A antagonist for the treatment of Parkinson's disease. Expert Rev Neurother. 2021;21(3):317-33.
16. Hauser RA, Hsu A, Kell S, Espay AJ, Sethi K, Stacy M, et al.; IPX066 ADVANCE-PD investigators. Extended-release carbidopa-levodopa (IPX066)

compared with immediate-release carbidopa-levodopa in patients with Parkinson's disease and motor fluctuations: a phase 3 randomised, double-blind trial. Lancet Neurol. 2013;12(4): 346-56.

17. Swope DM. Rapid treatment of "wearing off" in Parkinson's disease. Neurology. 2004;62(6 Suppl 4):S27-31.
18. LeWitt PA, Hauser RA, Pahwa R, Isaacson SH, Fernandez HH, Lew M, et al.; SPAN-PD Study Investigators. Safety and efficacy of CVT-301 (levodopa inhalation powder) on motor function during off periods in patients with Parkinson's disease: a randomised, double-blind, placebo-controlled phase 3 trial. Lancet Neurol. 2019;18(2):145-54.
19. Glenardi G, Handayani T, Barus J, Mangkuliguna G. Inhaled Levodopa (CVT-301) for the Treatment of Parkinson Disease: A Systematic Review and Meta-analysis of Randomized Controlled Trials. Neurol Clin Pract. 2022;12(2):139-48.
20. Chen JJ, Obering C. A review of intermittent subcutaneous apomorphine injections for the rescue management of motor fluctuations associated with advanced Parkinson's disease. Clin Ther. 2005;27(11):1710-24.
21. Cereda E, Barichella M, Pedrolli C, Pezzoli G. Low-protein and protein-redistribution diets for Parkinson's disease patients with motor fluctuations: a systematic review. Mov Disord. 2010;25(13):2021-34.
22. Rascol O, Fabbri M, Poewe W. Amantadine in the treatment of Parkinson's disease and other movement disorders. Lancet Neurol. 2021;20(12):1048-56.
23. Friedman JH. Clozapine Is Severely Underused in Parkinson's Disease Patients. Mov Disord Clin Pract. 2022;9(8):1021-4.
24. Olanow CW, Kieburtz K, Odin P, Espay AJ, Standaert DG, Fernandez HH, et al.; LCIG Horizon Study Group. Continuous intrajejunal infusion of levodopa-carbidopa intestinal gel for patients with advanced Parkinson's disease: a randomised, controlled, double-blind, double-dummy study. Lancet Neurol. 2014;13(2):141-9.
25. Sakakibara R, Uchiyama T, Yamanishi T, Kishi M. Genitourinary dysfunction in Parkinson's disease. Mov Disord. 2010;25(1):2-12.
26. Cho SY, Jeong SJ, Lee S, Kim J, Lee SH, Choo MS, et al. Mirabegron for treatment of overactive bladder symptoms in patients with Parkinson's disease: A double-blind, randomized placebo-controlled trial (Parkinson's Disease Overactive bladder Mirabegron, PaDoMi Study). Neurourol Urodyn. 2021;40(1):286-94.
27. Lamotte G, Lenka A. Orthostatic Hypotension in Parkinson Disease: What Is New? Neurol Clin Pract. 2022;12(5):e112-e115.
28. Safarpour D, Stover N, Shprecher DR, Hamedani AG, Pfeiffer RF, Parkman HP, et al.; Other Non-motor Features Working Group of the Parkinson Study Group. Consensus practice recommendations for management of gastrointestinal dysfunction in Parkinson disease. Parkinsonism Relat Disord. 2024;124:106982.
29. Mehta S, Lal V. Treatment of sialorrhea in Parkinson's disease. Ann Mov Disord. 2022;5(3): 153-8.
30. Goldman JG, Weintraub D. Advances in the treatment of cognitive impairment in Parkinson's disease. Mov Disord. 2015;30(11):1471-89.
31. Takamiya A, Seki M, Kudo S, Yoshizaki T, Nakahara J, Mimura M, et al. Electroconvulsive Therapy for Parkinson's Disease: A Systematic Review and Meta-Analysis. Mov Disord. 2021;36(1):50-8.
32. Yunusa I, Rashid N, Seyedin R, Paratane D, Rajagopalan K. Comparative Efficacy, Safety, and Acceptability of Pimavanserin and Other Atypical Antipsychotics for Parkinson's Disease Psychosis: Systematic Review and Network Meta-Analysis. J Geriatr Psychiatry Neurol. 2023;36(5):417-32.
33. Rissardo JP, Durante Í, Sharon I, Fornari Caprara AL. Pimavanserin and Parkinson's Disease Psychosis: A Narrative Review. Brain Sci. 2022;12(10):1286.
34. Nonnekes J, Snijders AH, Nutt JG, Deuschl G, Giladi N, Bloem BR. Freezing of gait: a practical approach to management. Lancet Neurol. 2015;14(7): 768-78.
35. Chang FC, Tsui DS, Mahant N, Wolfe N, Kim SD, Ha AD, et al. 24 h Levodopa-carbidopa intestinal gel may reduce falls and "unresponsive" freezing of gait in Parkinson's disease. Parkinsonism Relat Disord. 2015;21(3):317-20.
36. Cui CK, Lewis SJG. Future Therapeutic Strategies for Freezing of Gait in Parkinson's Disease. Front Hum Neurosci. 2021;15:741918.

CHAPTER 3

Device-assisted Therapies for Parkinson's Disease

Abhishek Vaingankar, Divya M Radhakrishnan, Roopa Rajan

ABSTRACT

Parkinson's disease (PD) in the mid stages is characterized by the development of motor complications including motor fluctuations and dyskinesias. Several advanced therapies are currently available to help patients who experience troublesome motor complications despite optimal medical therapy. These include surgical strategies such as deep brain stimulation, magnetic resonance-guided high-frequency-focused ultrasound lesioning, and radiofrequency ablation, as well as infusion therapies—continuous subcutaneous apomorphine infusion, intrajejunal levodopa infusions, and subcutaneous foslevodopa/foscarbidopa infusion. While all these are approved therapies that offer good control of motor symptoms in general, the specific benefits and risks vary. In this chapter, we will review the salient features of each therapy and the approach to making individualized and patient centered decisions regarding the initiation of these therapies.

Keywords: Neuromodulation, Parkinson's disease, Device assisted therapies, Advanced PD, DBS, CSAI, Infusion therapies, MRgFUS.

INTRODUCTION

The prevalence of Parkinson's disease (PD) doubled in the past 25 years.[1] Current estimates suggest that, in 2019, PD resulted in 5.8 million disability-adjusted life years, an increase of 81% since 2000, and caused 329,000 deaths, an increase of over 100% since 2000. PD is unique among other neurodegenerative diseases for its duration, which can span decades. While the motor symptoms of PD can be managed well with medications in the early stages of the disease, with the passage of time, persons living with PD start experiencing troublesome motor complications. Current standard of care for motor complications that remain uncontrolled despite best medical therapy includes several device-assisted advanced therapies, including deep brain stimulation (DBS), continuous subcutaneous apomorphine infusion (CSAI) and MR-guided focused ultrasound (MRgFUS) **(Flowchart 1)**. In this chapter, we will review important concepts involved in offering these advanced therapies in PD.

WHEN CAN DEVICE-AIDED THERAPIES BE OFFERED TO PATIENTS WITH PD?

Device-assisted therapies are generally considered in the mid-stages of PD, after the onset of motor complications, but before the appearance of clinically significant cognitive

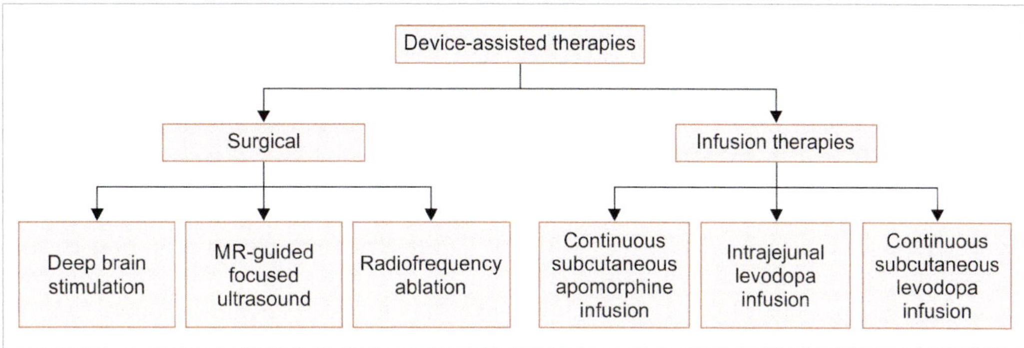

FLOWCHART 1: Device-assisted therapies in Parkinson's disease (PD).

dysfunction, medication refractory gait and axial symptoms and autonomic dysfunction that are considered markers of advanced disease. Motor complications may be noted in the form of either motor fluctuations (wearing off, delayed on, unpredictable off, and sudden off) or medication-induced dyskinesias. While current evidence does not support the use of advanced therapies very early in the disease course, before the onset of motor complications, there is no consensus as to how long medical strategies need to be tried before considering device-assisted therapies. Generally, advanced therapies are not considered prior to 4 years of disease duration, primarily to avoid inadvertently offering these treatments to patients with atypical parkinsonism. Patients with motor complications leading to functional decline [worsening of quality of life (QoL), reduced independence in daily life activities, and affecting professional activities], despite optimal medical therapy merit evaluation for advanced therapies.[2-4] The "5-2-1 criteria" (≥ five times daily oral levodopa, ≥ 2 daily hours with off symptoms or ≥ 1 daily hour with troublesome dyskinesia) may be useful as a screening tool to identify such patients.[5-8] Medication refractory tremor, even in the absence of motor complications or dyskinesias, may also benefit from an early consideration of device-assisted therapies, particularly surgical ones.

DEEP BRAIN STIMULATION

Deep brain stimulation was approved for the management of PD in 2002. Long-term efficacy is established for PD with documented improvement in the cardinal motor symptoms of PD and motor complications, such as motor fluctuations and dyskinesias.[9] Despite the widespread use of DBS, the mechanisms underpinning its therapeutic efficacy remain unclear. Hypothetical mechanisms of action include disruption of the abnormal synchronized activity in the basal ganglia circuits and normalization of aberrant cortical plasticity.[10] It is important to note that DBS is a symptom controlling therapy that has no disease modifying effects and cannot change or reverse the progressive disease course.

Deep brain stimulation entails continuous, high frequency electrical stimulation of a target nucleus with the help of strategically placed intracranial electrodes, connected to an implanted pulse generator (IPG) that is located subcutaneously in the chest wall.[11] Accurate implantation of electrodes into the target nucleus is achieved by a three-pronged strategy consisting of (1) direct or indirect visualization of the target nucleus on cranial MRI and stereotactic localization, (2) analysis of microelectrode recordings (MERs) obtained intraoperatively to identify the borders of the target nucleus, and (3) macrostimulation and clinical assessment of benefits and adverse events during the surgery.[12] The electrode implantation is usually performed through an awake craniotomy, under local anesthesia, while the IPG is implanted under general anesthesia.[13] Currently several types of IPGs are available, including rechargeable, nonrechargeable devices, and those with capabilities to record local field potentials from the target nucleus while concomitantly delivering stimulation.[13,14] DBS lead designs have also evolved over the years, to facilitate directional or tailored stimulation based on the needs of individual patients.[15]

The two most commonly used targets for DBS in PD are the subthalamic nucleus (STN) and globus pallidus internus (GPi).[16] DBS at the caudal zona incerta and pedunculopontine nucleus still remain experimental.[17-20] Both the commonly used targets appear to be similarly effective, albeit with important differences.[21] Overall, STN-DBS tends to be preferred for control of resting tremor and rigidity, allowing for a greater reduction in dopaminergic medication dose (50–70%), and subsequent reduction in dyskinesias. However, STN stimulation may potentially lead to worsening of certain nonmotor symptoms, including apathy, depression, impulsivity, verbal fluency, executive function, and freezing of gait.[22,23] It is unknown whether these undesirable effects are related to the drastic medication reduction following STN stimulation, or a stimulation induced effect. On the other hand, GPi DBS is particularly useful in controlling dyskinesias, and in patients with off time dystonia. GPi stimulation results in lesser medication reduction compared to STN and lesser cognitive, mood and gait dysfunction.[24] Earlier concerns about less robust tremor control and higher frequency of revision surgeries in GPi DBS do not seem to be validated by the larger, more recent randomized trials comparing the two targets. Hence, especially for elderly patients with borderline cognitive deficits and gait impairment, GPi is increasingly the preferred target.

Patient Selection for Deep Brain Stimulation

Deep brain stimulation is beneficial to patients with established PD, experiencing motor fluctuations and/or dyskinesias that remain troublesome despite the best medical therapy. Diagnosis of atypical parkinsonism is the only absolute contraindication to DBS **(Table 1)**. There is no well-defined cutoff age

TABLE 1: Inclusion and exclusion criteria for deep brain stimulation (DBS).

Inclusion criteria	Absolute exclusion criteria
Diagnosis of established Parkinson's disease (PD) > 4 years duration	Diagnosis of atypical parkinsonism
Troublesome motor fluctuations or dyskinesias despite optimal medical therapy	Relative exclusion criteria
	Clinically significant cognitive impairment/dementia
	Medication refractory axial/gait disturbances
	Symptomatic and severe autonomic dysfunction
	Uncontrolled psychiatric comorbidities— depression, suicidal ideation, hallucinations, etc. (need to be treated prior to surgery)
	Advanced age (no absolute cut-off, caution is advised >75–80 years)
	Poor social support

above which DBS is not considered, but long-term outcomes are generally less robust in the older age groups, while the surgical risks are higher.[25-29]

Levodopa responsiveness is the best predictor of motor outcomes after DBS.[9] Levodopa response assessment involves withdrawal of PD medication for 12 hours (defined off) and assessment of motor symptoms with a standardized scale, such as the Unified Parkinson's Disease Rating Scale (UPDRS) or the Movement Disorder Society-UPDRS (MDS-UPDRS). After the baseline assessment in the off state, patients receive a dose of levodopa/carbidopa. The dose used varies from center to center, ranging from the patient's habitual morning dose to 120–150% of their habitual morning dose.[9] While an improvement of at least 33% is considered levodopa responsive, best candidates for surgery generally have levodopa responsiveness scores upward of 50%.[30,31] A notable exception to this rule is the presence of levodopa resistant tremor which may improve with stimulation, even if it does not respond to medications.[12] The cardinal motor symptoms of PD—rest tremor, bradykinesia, rigidity, and dyskinesias improve significantly with DBS, resulting in improved QoL and activities of daily living. Freezing of gait and imbalance, especially when medication refractory, do not generally improve and may worsen with time as part of disease progression. So also cognitive impairment and hence, these are considered relative contraindications to DBS surgery. Speech quality may worsen postoperatively, though this may be mitigated to a certain extent by programming parameter adjustments.[32] DBS is primarily performed for control of motor symptoms; however, certain nonmotor symptoms such as pain, constipation, and sleep quality may improve after DBS. Verbal fluency is known to decline after STN-DBS, though it does not usually result in clinically significant cognitive impairments. Other nonmotor symptoms such as mood (depression or mania), anxiety, and apathy may worsen, often transiently and more so after STN-DBS.[33] Impulse control disorders (ICDs) have a double-edged relationship with DBS, preexisting ICDs often improve with dopaminergic reduction postoperatively, while new onset ICDs may develop in a few.[34]

BOX 1: Preoperative evaluation for deep brain stimulation (DBS) surgical candidates.

- Clinical evaluation by movement disorder specialist neurologist for diagnostic confirmation
- Levodopa response assessment
- Comprehensive cognitive evaluation—at minimum, a detailed screening tool such as Addenbrooke's cognitive examination (ACE) and lobar assessments for frontal lobe
- Neuropsychiatric evaluation and screening for depression, mania, anxiety, hallucinations, impulse control disorders
- Surgical risk evaluation and preanesthetic check up
- Contrast enhanced MRI brain including sequences used for DBS planning [e.g., Fast Gray Matter Acquisition T1 Inversion Recovery (FGATIR)]

Surgical risks in DBS include perioperative complications such as intracranial hemorrhage (2–3%), implant infections (2–3%), and anesthetic risks. Lead breakage and migration are unusually encountered. Sudden cessation of stimulation due to IPG depletion or removal can result in a life-threatening malignant STN-DBS withdrawal syndrome, akin to neuroleptic malignant syndrome. A comprehensive multidisciplinary evaluation is mandatory in the preoperative selection to assess the above features and make an individualized decision **(Box 1)**.

MR-GUIDED FOCUSED ULTRASOUND

MR-guided focused ultrasound ablation is a recently introduced technique for minimally invasive lesioning of target nuclei in the brain. Unilateral MRgFUS thalamotomy and pallidotomy are the Food and Drug Administration (FDA) approved for treatment of PD. The technology involves using a helmet-based phased array transducer to pass ultrasound beams through an intact skull to a common focal point, under MRI guidance. The subsequent coagulative necrosis results in therapeutic effects akin to lesioning.[35]

Current approval is limited to unilateral procedures for ventral intermediate (VIM) ablation in tremor dominant PD and pallidotomy in patients with motor fluctuations and dyskinesias. A double-blind randomized controlled trial (RCT) in 27 patients with tremor dominant PD targeting the VIM nucleus of the thalamus showed significant improvement in the tremor at 3 months. Side effects included mild hemiparesis, perioral paresthesias, and ataxia.[35-37] Randomized trial of unilateral MRgFUS ablation of the GPi showed benefit in controlling PD motor features and in reducing dyskinesias. Adverse events included dysarthria and gait disturbances, majority of which resolved by 12 months.[36] Studies on additional targets such as the STN, pallidothalamic tract, and for bilateral procedures are ongoing.

Advantages of MRgFUS include its non-invasive nature, avoiding the need for both craniotomy and general anesthesia, which is particularly useful for individuals with advanced age and surgical risks. It also avoids the use of an implanted device and multiple programming visits for titration of effects. The most important limitation is that safety of bilateral procedures is not yet established; bilateral lesioning using other modalities, such as radiofrequency (RF) ablation has resulted in high incidence of postoperative dysarthria, dysphagia, and axial symptoms which limit the overall gains in QoL. Since it is a lesioning procedure, postoperative changes cannot be made to control for these issues. Higher skull density ratios in Asian patients may also be a limitation to the passage of ultrasound beams. Being a newer technology, long-term results beyond the initial years are as yet unknown.

RADIOFREQUENCY LESIONING

Radiofrequency lesioning studies were among the earliest therapies offered for PD since the 1930s. With the advent of levodopa, lesioning surgeries fell out of favor and further reduced in popularity after DBS became widely available.[38] Nevertheless, RF lesioning of the pallidum has been studied in observational studies and small RCTs. Unilateral pallidotomy results in about 20–30% reduction in the off time motor symptoms and is particularly effective for drug-induced dyskinesias and dystonia. Effects on QoL are not known. Bilateral pallidotomy procedures are now largely abandoned due to a higher risk of permanent dysarthria and dysphagia. Advantages of pallidotomy over DBS include the rapidity of onset of effect, avoidance of implant and associated risks such as infections, lack of requirement for programming and low cost.[39] Disadvantages include inability to perform bilateral procedures and risk of permanent side effects. Advances in neuroimaging techniques and studies on alternative targets, such as the pallidothalamic tract may increase the utility of this technique in the future.

CONTINUOUS SUBCUTANEOUS APOMORPHINE INFUSION

Apomorphine is a dopamine D1 and D2 receptor agonist with rapid onset and offset of action, available in injectable form.[40] Apomorphine can be delivered as a continuous subcutaneous infusion during awake hours, via a dose regulator external pump.

The indications to consider CSAI are similar to that for any advanced therapy in PD. However, it is generally considered in two situations: (1) Patients in whom surgical therapies like DBS are contraindicated due to high surgical risks or advanced cognitive and gait deficits or (2) as part of best medical therapy in patients who like to avoid or delay DBS.[41] CSAI received marketing approval following a single international multicentric, randomized trial (the TOLEDO study) which showed a >2-hour reduction in daily off time after 12 weeks of treatment in >50% of patients, with a mean reduction in off time of 1.89 hours and an increase in the on time without problematic dyskinesia by 1.97 hours compared to placebo.[42] However, the effect of CSAI on the QoL was not studied in this trial.[43-45]

Prior to initiation of CSAI an apomorphine response test is required to confirm the efficacy and dose required. In the off medication state, response to apomorphine subcutaneous injection is assessed in increments of 1 mg, till a maximum of 7 mg (up to 10 mg in partial responders). An improvement in UPDRS/MDS-UPDRS score of 30% is considered responsive. Responders may subsequently be initiated on continuous infusion. Typically, the infusion is started at rates of 0.5–1 mg/hour with gradual increments over several hour/days to reach optimal symptom control along with reduction of concomitant medications. It may take up to 3 weeks to reach optimal doses and the routine doses are in the range of 2–7 mg/hour for majority of patients. The infusion is usually provided during awake hours (10–16 hours/day) except in unusual circumstances when required for severe nocturnal symptoms. Tolerance may occur with long term, continuous use.

The most common adverse effect with CSAI is nodular skin eruptions (54.8% of patients on CSAI in the TOLEDO study), rotating the site of infusion is essential to reduce these.[46] Other device-related issues include infections, breakage, etc. Nausea and vomiting may be limiting side effects, and patients are premedicated with antiemetics (domperidone) at the initiation of treatment. Other medication-related side effects include somnolence, hypotension, worsening of dyskinesias, hallucinations, hemolytic anemia, and QT interval prolongation on electrocardiogram (ECG). These need to be monitored throughout the use of therapy.[47]

INTRAJEJUNAL LEVODOPA INFUSION

Levodopa-carbidopa Intestinal Gel Therapy

Levodopa-carbidopa intestinal gel (LCIG) therapy involves administering a gel suspension of levodopa/carbidopa monohydrate (20 mg/mL and 5 mg/mL; 4:1 ratio) to the patient's small intestine via a portable pump and a tube inserted through a percutaneous endoscopic gastrojejunostomy (PEG-J).[40] By delivering the drugs directly to the jejunum, the system aims to bypass delayed gastric motility in individuals with advanced PD.[48] Usually a 16-hour infusion is administered to patients while they are awake, though A 24-hour infusion maybe used for patients with severe nocturnal or early morning "off" symptoms, or disabling dyskinesia caused by flushing the tube before stopping the LCIG pump.[49] The LCIG daily dose includes a morning bolus, a continuous dose, and an extra bolus if necessary.[50] A typical morning dose comprises 100–200 mg of levodopa, which takes 10–30 minutes to reach a therapeutic plasma concentration. The continuous dose of levodopa, ranging from 20 to 200 mg/h, is infused throughout the day and adjusted based on symptomatology.[50]

Many clinical trials have confirmed the safety and efficacy of LCIG, leading to its FDA approval in 2015.[51-53] LCIG treatment has proven to improve the health-related QoL in individuals with advanced PD.[54-56] Patients who undergo LCIG treatment experience a reduction in off time and an increase in on time without bothersome dyskinesias.[53,57,58] LCIG therapy can improve various nonmotor symptoms, such as sleep, anxiety, depression, hallucinations, and ICDs.[59,60] Adverse effects associated with levodopa/carbidopa include dyskinesias, psychoses, weight loss, dopamine dysregulation syndrome, orthostatic hypotension, and polyneuropathy. The device itself can lead to complications such as local infection, displacement, ulcers, pneumoperitoneum, and ileus.[61,62] The occurrence of peripheral neuropathy during LCIG treatment is a subject of controversy. It is not known if the neuropathy is directly caused by the LCIG treatment itself, the high doses of levodopa used, or if it results from the underlying disease.[63] It is advised that patients receiving LCIG therapy undergo periodic electrophysiological evaluations and tests to detect vitamin B12 and folic acid deficiency.[64,65] Treatment with catechol-O-methyltransferase inhibitors has been shown to lower the risk of polyneuropathy in patients treated with levodopa.[66]

The LCIG therapy is most appropriate for individuals with advanced PD, experiencing severe motor fluctuations or troublesome dyskinesia, who cannot undergo DBS or prefer a less invasive treatment.[12,67] Patients who have a poor response to levodopa, pronounced dementia, inability to handle the infusion pump, or contraindications for abdominal surgery may not be suitable for LCIG therapy.[50]

Levodopa/Entacapone/Carbidopa Intestinal Gel Therapy

The levodopa-entacapone-carbidopa intestinal gel (LECIG) is a recent addition to the therapeutic options for PD with motor fluctuations.[40] The presence of entacapone (20 mg/mL) in LECIG, along with levodopa (20 mg/mL) and carbidopa (5 mg/mL), improves the bioavailability of levodopa by reducing its peripheral metabolism.[68] This allows a lower daily levodopa doses while still achieving a stable therapeutic plasma level. LECIG infusion is compatible with the PEG-J system used in LCIG infusion and features a smaller cartridge and pump system.[69] The clinical efficacy of LECIG is similar to LCIG in improving motor symptoms.[70] By minimizing the exposure to harmful levodopa metabolites, LECIG may also potentially reduce the risk of polyneuropathy associated with LCIG.[71] However, studies have not consistently proven that LECIG is superior in terms of safety, continuation rates, and reduced levodopa doses compared to LCIG.[72] Various European countries have authorized the use of LECIG infusion for advanced PD.[71]

CONTINUOUS SUBCUTANEOUS LEVODOPA INFUSION

Foslevodopa (LDp) and foscarbidopa (CDp) are prodrugs of levodopa and carbidopa which are converted into their active forms in the liver, thus ensuring a continuous and stable supply of levodopa and carbidopa.[73] This has emerged as a promising therapy for advanced PD.[74-76] BouNDless, a phase 3, randomized, double-blind, double-dummy, multicenter trial tested the efficacy of this infusion in patients of PD aged 30 years or more who experienced a mean off time of at least 2.5 h/day over 3 consecutive days (≥2 hours each day) unamenable to drug manipulation.[77] Treatment with subcutaneous LDp/CDp provided an additional 1.72 hours [95% confidence interval (CI) 1.08–2.36] of on time without troublesome dyskinesia compared with oral levodopa-carbidopa. Subcutaneous infusion of 700/35 mg LDp/CDp over 24 hours provides comparable levodopa exposures to LCIG infusion 350/87.5 mg administered over 16 hours, followed by two 100/25 mg levodopa-carbidopa oral doses.[73]

Infusion site reactions are common adverse effects.[76] Frequent injection site rotation may help mitigate this adverse reaction. Gastrointestinal (GI) side effects like nausea occurred at a higher frequency than on oral levodopa-carbidopa. Long-term safety and tolerability with this formulation is yet to be examined.[76] This therapy is currently approved in the EU and Canada but is yet to receive the FDA approval.[78-80]

OTHER DEVICE-ASSISTED THERAPIES IN DEVELOPMENT

Spinal cord stimulation (SCS) is an approved therapy for medication refractory chronic pain. Its efficacy to improve gait, specifically freezing of gait and imbalance in patients with PD, is being studied and small studied have shown promise in improving gait related QoL with an acceptable risk profile.[81] Transcranial magnetic stimulation (TMS) is noninvasive technique to modulate the cortical plasticity, several studies have assessed the utility of TMS in motor and nonmotor symptoms in PD. High frequency (10 Hz) TMS to the dorsolateral prefrontal cortex is approved by the FDA for major depression. While small studies using different protocols and targets have shown beneficial effects on dyskinesias, gait, rigidity, and other symptoms of PD, no consensus exists on optimal target and paradigm for stimulation. Similarly, a meta-analysis of studies on transcranial direct current stimulation (tDCS) did not show consistent benefits.[82] The use of these therapies (TMS, tCDS, and SCS) remain investigational and they are best considered in a clinical trial setting.

CHOOSING AMONG THE DEVICE-ASSISTED THERAPIES

With the repertoire of available options, an individual patient may be eligible for one or more of the device-assisted therapies. There are no head-to-head trials among most of the advanced therapies. A network meta-analysis that compared DBS, CSAI, LCIG, pallidotomy, and medical therapy identified that STN-DBS, GPi-DBS, and intrajejunal levodopa infusion (IJLI) led to better QoL than medical therapy alone. STN-DBS alleviated more patient and clinician relevant outcomes and was adjudged as having the highest probability of improving QoL, followed by GPi-DBS and IJLI.[12] While CSAI improved motor outcomes, it did not improve activities of daily living and its effect on QoL was not known. The most recent guidelines from the European Federation of Neurological Societies (EFNS)/MDS reflect these findings, and provide guidance toward choosing among the options. The choice of therapy has to be made considering the benefits, limitations, risks, and expectations in each individual **(Table 2)**.[83,84]

TABLE 2: How to choose among therapies—examples for individualized decision-making.[83]

Patient profile	Intervention	Rationale	Comments
PD with prominent motor fluctuations	• STN-DBS or GPi-DBS • Other options include LCIG and CSAI	Multiple studies have shown improvements in motor fluctuations and dyskinesias with DBS	Long-term benefits with CSAI and LCIG remain understudied
PD with early fluctuations	STN-DBS, CSAI	The EarlyStim trial showed benefit of STN-DBS soon after the onset of motor fluctuations[84]	CSAI may be offered as part of best medical therapy for patients who are not keen for surgery

Continued

Continued

Patient profile	Intervention	Rationale	Comments
Patients with prominent tremor	STN-DBS, GPi-DBS or MRgFUS	In view of established long-term efficacy and possibility of newer symptoms appearing in future, DBS should be the first option for such patients, especially younger patients	MRgFUS thalamotomy may be an option in patients with asymmetric tremor but long-term data is not available, maybe beneficial in elderly with multiple comorbidities and high surgical risks
PD with cognitive impairment	GPi-DBS, IJLI, CSAI, MRgFUS thalamotomy for unilateral tremor	GPI maybe preferred over STN in patients with early cognitive impairment. Risk of lower therapeutic benefit needs to be counseled. For patients with more advanced cognitive impairment, IJLI or CSAI maybe more suitable	Lack of controlled studies in MCI or dementia patients

(CSAI: continuous subcutaneous apomorphine infusion; DBS: deep brain stimulation; GPi: globus pallidus internus; IJLI: intrajejunal levodopa infusion; LCIG: levodopa-carbidopa intestinal gel; MCI: mild cognitive impairment; MRgFUS: MR-guided focused ultrasound; PD: Parkinson's disease; STN: subthalamic nucleus)

CONCLUSION

Device aided therapies in Parkinson's Disease represent an ever evolving landscape and have been definitively shown to improve quality of life in carefully chosen patients. Given an array of options to choose from, device aided therapies may be selected on the basis of patient profile and anticipated adverse effects. Multidisciplinary management, patient counselling and a sound technical expertise are necessary to achieve good outcomes.

REFERENCES

1. GBD 2016 Neurology Collaborators. Global, regional, and national burden of neurological disorders, 1990–2016: a systematic analysis for the Global Burden of Disease Study 2016. Lancet Neurol. 2019;18(5):459-480.
2. Titova N, Martinez-Martin P, Katunina E, Chaudhuri KR. Advanced Parkinson's or "complex phase" Parkinson's disease? Re-evaluation is needed. J Neural Transm. 2017;124(12):1529-37.
3. Sesar Á, Fernández-Pajarín G, Ares B, Castro A. Do we need to redefine the advanced stage in Parkinson's disease? Revista Mexicana de Neurociencia. 2021;22(4).
4. Auffret M, Weiss D, Stocchi F, Vérin M, Jost WH. Access to device-aided therapies in advanced Parkinson's disease: navigating clinician biases, patient preference, and prognostic uncertainty. J Neural Transm. 2023;130(11):1411-32.
5. Aldred J, Anca-Herschkovitsch M, Antonini A, Bajenaru O, Bergmann L, Bourgeois P, et al. Application of the '5-2-1' Screening Criteria in Advanced Parkinson's Disease: Interim Analysis of DUOGLOBE. Neurodegener Dis Manag. 2020;10(5):309-23.
6. Santos-García D, de Deus Fonticoba T, Suárez Castro E, Aneiros Díaz A, McAfee D. 5-2-1 Criteria: A Simple Screening Tool for Identifying Advanced PD Patients Who Need an Optimization of Parkinson's Treatment. Parkinsons Dis. 2020;2020:1-6.
7. Martinez-Martin P, Kulisevsky J, Mir P, Tolosa E, García-Delgado P, Luquin MR. Validation of a simple screening tool for early diagnosis of advanced Parkinson's disease in daily practice: the CDEPA questionnaire. NPJ Parkinsons Dis. 2018;4(1):20.

8. Antonini A, Stoessl AJ, Kleinman LS, Skalicky AM, Marshall TS, Sail KR, et al. Developing consensus among movement disorder specialists on clinical indicators for identification and management of advanced Parkinson's disease: a multi-country Delphi-panel approach. Curr Med Res Opin. 2018;34(12):2063-73.
9. Aquino CH de, Moscovich M, Marinho MM, Barcelos LB, Felício AC, Halverson M, et al. Fundamentals of deep brain stimulation for Parkinson's disease in clinical practice: part 1. Arq Neuropsiquiatr. 2024;82(4):1-9.
10. Ashkan K, Rogers P, Bergman H, Ughratdar I. Insights into the mechanisms of deep brain stimulation. Nat Rev Neurol. 2017;13(9):548-54.
11. Lee D, Dallapiazza R, De Vloo P, Lozano A. Current surgical treatments for Parkinson's disease and potential therapeutic targets. Neural Regen Res. 2018;13(8):1342.
12. Rajan R, Skorvanek M, Magocova V, Siddiqui J, AlSinaidi OA, Shinawi HM, et al. Neuromodulation Options and Patient Selection for Parkinson's Disease. Neurol India. 2020;68(8):S170-8.
13. Stewart CDM, Eljamel S. Prediction of implantable pulse generator longevity in deep brain stimulation: limitations and possible solutions in clinical practice. Stereotact Funct Neurosurg. 2011;89(5):299-304.
14. Anheim M, Fraix V, Chabardès S, Krack P, Benabid AL, Pollak P. Lifetime of Itrel II pulse generators for subthalamic nucleus stimulation in Parkinson's disease. Mov Disord. 2007;22(16):2436-9.
15. Schüpbach WMM, Chabardes S, Matthies C, Pollo C, Steigerwald F, Timmermann L, et al. Directional leads for deep brain stimulation: Opportunities and challenges. Mov Disord. 2017;32(10):1371-5.
16. Strauss I, Kalia SK, Lozano AM. Where are we with surgical therapies for Parkinson's disease? Parkinsonism Relat Disord. 2014;20 Suppl 1:S187-91.
17. Weiss D, Walach M, Meisner C, Fritz M, Scholten M, Breit S, et al. Nigral stimulation for resistant axial motor impairment in Parkinson's disease? A randomized controlled trial. Brain. 2013;136(7):2098-108.
18. Khan S, Javed S, Mooney L, White P, Plaha P, Whone A, et al. Clinical outcomes from bilateral versus unilateral stimulation of the pedunculopontine nucleus with and without concomitant caudal zona incerta region stimulation in Parkinson's disease. Br J Neurosurg. 2012;26(5):722-5.
19. Stefani A, Lozano AM, Peppe A, Stanzione P, Galati S, Tropepi D, et al. Bilateral deep brain stimulation of the pedunculopontine and subthalamic nuclei in severe Parkinson's disease. Brain. 2007;130(Pt 6):1596-607.
20. Khan S, Mooney L, Plaha P, Javed S, White P, Whone AL, et al. Outcomes from stimulation of the caudal zona incerta and pedunculopontine nucleus in patients with Parkinson's disease. Br J Neurosurg. 2011;25(2):273-80.
21. Lukins TR, Tisch S, Jonker B. The latest evidence on target selection in deep brain stimulation for Parkinson's disease. J Clin Neurosci. 2014;21(1): 22-7.
22. Mansouri A, Taslimi S, Badhiwala JH, Witiw CD, Nassiri F, Odekerken VJJ, et al. Deep brain stimulation for Parkinson's disease: meta-analysis of results of randomized trials at varying lengths of follow-up. J Neurosurg. 2018;128(4):1199-213.
23. Hariz MI, Rehncrona S, Quinn NP, Speelman JD, Wensing C. Multicenter study on deep brain stimulation in Parkinson's disease: an independent assessment of reported adverse events at 4 years. Mov Disord. 2008;23(3):416-21.
24. Odekerken VJJ, van Laar T, Staal MJ, Mosch A, Hoffmann CF, Nijssen PC, et al. Subthalamic nucleus versus globus pallidus bilateral deep brain stimulation for advanced Parkinson's disease (NSTAPS study): a randomised controlled trial. Lancet Neurol. 2013;12(1):37-44.
25. Lang AE, Widner H. Deep brain stimulation for Parkinson's disease: patient selection and evaluation. Mov Disord. 2002;17 Suppl 3:S94-101.
26. Katz M, Kilbane C, Rosengard J, Alterman RL, Tagliati M. Referring patients for deep brain stimulation: an improving practice. Arch Neurol. 2011;68(8):1027-32.
27. DeLong MR, Huang KT, Gallis J, Lokhnygina Y, Parente B, Hickey P, et al. Effect of advancing age on outcomes of deep brain stimulation for Parkinson disease. JAMA Neurol. 2014;71(10):1290-5.
28. Bronstein JM, Tagliati M, Alterman RL, Lozano AM, Volkmann J, Stefani A, et al. Deep Brain Stimulation for Parkinson Disease: An Expert Consensus and Review of Key Issues. Arch Neurol. 2011;68(2):165.
29. Russmann H, Ghika J, Villemure JG, Robert B, Bogousslavsky J, Burkhard PR, et al. Subthalamic nucleus deep brain stimulation in Parkinson disease patients over age 70 years. Neurology. 2004;63(10):1952-4.
30. Brandão P, Grippe TC, Modesto LC, Ferreira AGF, Silva FMD, Pereira FF, et al. Decisions about deep brain stimulation therapy in Parkinson's disease. Arq Neuropsiquiatr. 2018;76(6):411-20.

31. Rodriguez RL, Fernandez HH, Haq I, Okun MS. Pearls in patient selection for deep brain stimulation. Neurologist. 2007;13(5):253-60.
32. Rouaud T, Dondaine T, Drapier S, Haegelen C, Lallement F, Péron J, et al. Pallidal stimulation in advanced Parkinson's patients with contra-indications for subthalamic stimulation. Mov Disord. 2010;25(12):1839-46.
33. Chapuis S, Ouchchane L, Metz O, Gerbaud L, Durif F. Impact of the motor complications of Parkinson's disease on the quality of life. Mov Disord. 2005;20(2):224-30.
34. Fasano A, Romito LM, Daniele A, Piano C, Zinno M, Bentivoglio AR, et al. Motor and cognitive outcome in patients with Parkinson's disease 8 years after subthalamic implants. Brain. 2010;133(9):2664-76.
35. Verhagen Metman L, Monje MHG, Obeso JA, Martínez-Fernández R. Focused ultrasound therapy: Back to the future. Parkinsonism Relat Disord. 2024;121:106023.
36. Krishna V, Fishman PS, Eisenberg HM, Kaplitt M, Baltuch G, Chang JW, et al. Trial of Globus Pallidus Focused Ultrasound Ablation in Parkinson's Disease. N Engl J Med. 2023;388(8):683-93.
37. Stieglitz LH, Mahendran S, Oertel MF, Baumann CR. Bilateral Focused Ultrasound Pallidotomy for Parkinson-Related Facial Dyskinesia—A Case Report. Mov Disord Clin Pract. 2022;9(5):647-51.
38. Agrawal M, Garg K, Samala R, Rajan R, Singh M. A Scientometric Analysis of the 100 Most Cited Articles on Pallidotomy. Stereotact Funct Neurosurg. 2021;99(6):463-73.
39. Gross RE. What happened to posteroventral pallidotomy for Parkinson's disease and dystonia? Neurotherapeutics. 2008;5(2):281.
40. Antonini A, D'Onofrio V, Guerra A. Current and novel infusion therapies for patients with Parkinson's disease. J Neural Transm. 2023;130(11):1349-58.
41. Antonini A, Jenner P. Apomorphine infusion in advanced Parkinson disease. Nat Rev Neurol. 2018;14(12):693-4.
42. Katzenschlager R, Poewe W, Rascol O, Trenkwalder C, Deuschl G, Chaudhuri KR, et al. Apomorphine subcutaneous infusion in patients with Parkinson's disease with persistent motor fluctuations (TOLEDO): a multicentre, double-blind, randomised, placebo-controlled trial. Lancet Neurol. 2018;17(9):749-59.
43. Martinez-Martin P, Reddy P, Katzenschlager R, Antonini A, Todorova A, Odin P, et al. EuroInf: a multicenter comparative observational study of apomorphine and levodopa infusion in Parkinson's disease. Mov Disord. 2015;30(4):510-16.
44. Drapier S, Eusebio A, Degos B, Vérin M, Durif F, Azulay JP, et al. Quality of life in Parkinson's disease improved by apomorphine pump: the OPTIPUMP cohort study. J Neurol. 2016;263(6):1111-9.
45. Houvenaghel JF, Drapier S, Duprez J, Robert GH, Riou A, Drapier D, et al. Effects of continuous subcutaneous apomorphine infusion in Parkinson's disease without cognitive impairment on motor, cognitive, psychiatric symptoms and quality of life. J Neurol Sci. 2018;395:113-8.
46. Henriksen T, Katzenschlager R, Bhidayasiri R, Staines H, Lockhart D, Lees A. Practical use of apomorphine infusion in Parkinson's disease: lessons from the TOLEDO study and clinical experience. J Neural Transm. 2023;130(11):1475.
47. Metta V, Dhamija RK, Batzu L, Mrudula R, Kumar NSS, Falup-Pecurariu C, et al. Safety and tolerability of long-term apomorphine infusion in advanced Parkinson's disease: an Indian multi-center (APO-IND) experience. Sci Rep. 2023;13(1):18681.
48. Bestetti A, Capozza A, Lacerenza M, Manfredi L, Mancini F. Delayed Gastric Emptying in Advanced Parkinson Disease. Clin Nucl Med. 2017;42(2):83-7.
49. Thakkar S, Fung VSC, Merola A, Rollins M, Soileau MJ, Kovács N. 24-Hour Levodopa-Carbidopa Intestinal Gel: Clinical Experience and Practical Recommendations. CNS Drugs. 2021;35(2):137-49.
50. Timpka J, Nitu B, Datieva V, Odin P, Antonini A. Device-Aided Treatment Strategies in Advanced Parkinson's Disease. Int Rev Neurobiol. 2017;132:453-74.
51. Slevin JT, Fernandez HH, Zadikoff C, Hall C, Eaton S, Dubow J, et al. Long-term safety and maintenance of efficacy of levodopa-carbidopa intestinal gel: an open-label extension of the double-blind pivotal study in advanced Parkinson's disease patients. J Parkinsons Dis. 2015;5(1):165-74.
52. Fernandez HH, Standaert DG, Hauser RA, Lang AE, Fung VS, Klostermann F. et al. Levodopa-carbidopa intestinal gel in advanced Parkinson's disease: final 12-month, open-label results. Mov Disord. 2015;30(4):500-9.
53. Olanow CW, Kieburtz K, Odin P, Espay AJ, Standaert DG, Fernandez HH, et al. Continuous intrajejunal infusion of levodopa-carbidopa intestinal gel for patients with advanced Parkinson's disease: a randomised, controlled, double-blind, double-dummy study. Lancet Neurol. 2014;13(2):141-9.

54. Lopiano L, Modugno N, Marano P, Sensi M, Meco G, Solla P, et al. Motor and non-motor outcomes in patients with advanced Parkinson's disease treated with levodopa/carbidopa intestinal gel: final results of the GREENFIELD observational study. J Neurol. 2019;266(9):2164-76.
55. Juhász A, Aschermann Z, Ács P, Janszky J, Kovács M, Makkos A, et al. Levodopa/carbidopa intestinal gel can improve both motor and non-motor experiences of daily living in Parkinson's disease: An open-label study. Parkinsonism Relat Disord. 2017;37:79-86.
56. Antonini A, Poewe W, Chaudhuri KR, Jech R, Pickut B, Pirtošek Z, et al. Levodopa-carbidopa intestinal gel in advanced Parkinson's: Final results of the GLORIA registry. Parkinsonism Relat Disord. 2017;45:13-20.
57. Standaert DG, Aldred J, Anca-Herschkovitsch M, Bourgeois P, Cubo E, Davis TL, et al. DUOGLOBE: One-Year Outcomes in a Real-World Study of Levodopa Carbidopa Intestinal Gel for Parkinson's Disease. Mov Disord Clin Pract. 2021;8(7):1061-74.
58. Freire-Alvarez E, Kurča E, Lopez Manzanares L, Pekkonen E, Spanaki C, Vanni P, et al. Levodopa-Carbidopa Intestinal Gel Reduces Dyskinesia in Parkinson's Disease in a Randomized Trial. Mov Disord. 2021;36(11):2615-23.
59. Kamel WA, Al-Hashel JY. LCIG in treatment of non-motor symptoms in advanced Parkinson's disease: Review of literature. Brain Behav. 2020;10(9):e01757.
60. Antonini A, Yegin A, Preda C, Bergmann L, Poewe W. Global long-term study on motor and non-motor symptoms and safety of levodopa-carbidopa intestinal gel in routine care of advanced Parkinson's disease patients; 12-month interim outcomes. Parkinsonism Relat Disord. 2015;21(3):231-5.
61. Rus T, Premzl M, Križnar NZ, Kramberger MG, Rajnar R, Ocepek L, et al. Adverse effects of levodopa/carbidopa intrajejunal gel treatment: A single-center long-term follow-up study. Acta Neurol Scand. 2022;146(5):537-44.
62. Lang AE, Rodriguez RL, Boyd JT, Chouinard S, Zadikoff C, Espay AJ, et al. Integrated safety of levodopa-carbidopa intestinal gel from prospective clinical trials. Mov Disord. 2016;31(4):538-46.
63. Devigili G, Rinaldo S, Lettieri C, Eleopra R. Levodopa/carbidopa intestinal gel therapy for advanced Parkinson Disease: AN early toxic effect for small nerve fibers? Muscle Nerve. 2016;54(5):970-2.
64. Virhammar J, Nyholm D. Levodopa-carbidopa enteral suspension in advanced Parkinson's disease: clinical evidence and experience. Ther Adv Neurol Disord. 2017;10(3):171.
65. Taher J, Naranian T, Poon YY, Merola A, Mestre T, Suchowersky O, et al. Vitamins and Infusion of Levodopa-Carbidopa Intestinal Gel. Can J Neurol Sci. 2022;49(1):19-28.
66. Cossu G, Ceravolo R, Zibetti M, Arca R, Ricchi V, Paribello A, et al. Levodopa and neuropathy risk in patients with Parkinson disease: Effect of COMT inhibition. Parkinsonism Relat Disord. 2016;27: 81-4.
67. Antonini A, Pahwa R, Odin P, Isaacson SH, Merola A, Wang L, et al. Comparative Effectiveness of Device-Aided Therapies on Quality of Life and Off-Time in Advanced Parkinson's Disease: A Systematic Review and Bayesian Network Meta-analysis. CNS Drugs. 2022;36(12):1269-83.
68. Müller T. Catechol-O-methyltransferase inhibitors in Parkinson's disease. Drugs. 2015;75(2):157-74.
69. Öthman M, Widman E, Nygren I, Nyholm D. Initial Experience of the Levodopa–Entacapone–Carbidopa Intestinal Gel in Clinical Practice. J Pers Med. 2021;11(4):254.
70. Senek M, Nielsen EI, Nyholm D. Levodopa-entacapone-carbidopa intestinal gel in Parkinson's disease: A randomized crossover study. Mov Disord. 2017;32(2):283-6.
71. Nyholm D, Jost WH. Levodopa-entacapone-carbidopa intestinal gel infusion in advanced Parkinson's disease: real-world experience and practical guidance. Ther Adv Neurol Disord. 2022;15: 17562864221108018.
72. Viljaharju V, Mertsalmi T, Pauls KAM, Koivu M, Eerola-Rautio J, Udd M, et al. Levodopa-Entacapone-Carbidopa Intestinal Gel Treatment in Advanced Parkinson's Disease: A Single-Center Study of 30 Patients. Mov Disord Clin Pract. 2024;11(2):159-65.
73. Rosebraugh M, Liu W, Neenan M, Facheris MF. Foslevodopa/Foscarbidopa Is Well Tolerated and Maintains Stable Levodopa and Carbidopa Exposure Following Subcutaneous Infusion. J Parkinsons Dis. 2021;11(4):1695-702.
74. Aldred J, Freire-Alvarez E, Amelin AV, Antonini A, Bergmans B, Bergquist F, et al. Continuous Subcutaneous Foslevodopa/Foscarbidopa in Parkinson's Disease: Safety and Efficacy Results From a 12-Month, Single-Arm, Open-Label, Phase 3 Study. Neurol Ther. 2023;12(6):1937-58.
75. Rosebraugh M, Voight EA, Moussa EM, Jameel F, Lou X, Zhang GGZ, et al. Foslevodopa/

Foscarbidopa: A New Subcutaneous Treatment for Parkinson's Disease. Ann Neurol. 2021;90(1): 52-61.

76. Soileau MJ, Aldred J, Budur K, Fisseha N, Fung VS, Jeong A, et al. Safety and efficacy of continuous subcutaneous foslevodopa-foscarbidopa in patients with advanced Parkinson's disease: a randomised, double-blind, active-controlled, phase 3 trial. Lancet Neurol. 2022;21(12): 1099-109.
77. Espay AJ, Stocchi F, Pahwa R, Albanese A, Ellenbogen A, Ferreira JJ, et al. Safety and efficacy of continuous subcutaneous levodopa–carbidopa infusion (ND0612) for Parkinson's disease with motor fluctuations (BouNDless): a phase 3, randomised, double-blind, double-dummy, multicentre trial. Lancet Neurol. 2024;23(5): 465-76.
78. Canada's Drug Agency. Foslevodopa Foscarbidopa. [online] Available from https://www.cda-amc.ca/foslevodopa-foscarbidopa. [Last accessed August, 2024].
79. AbbVie. (2024). AbbVie Provides U.S. Regulatory Update on ABBV-951 (Foscarbidopa/Foslevodopa). [online] Available from https://news.abbvie.com/2024-06-25-AbbVie-Provides-U-S-Regulatory-Update-on-ABBV-951-Foscarbidopa-Foslevodopa. [Last accessed August, 2024].
80. AbbVie. (2024). AbbVie Launches PRODUODOPA® (foslevodopa/foscarbidopa) for People Living with Advanced Parkinson's Disease in the European Union. [online] Available from https://news.abbvie.com/2024-01-09-AbbVie-Launches-PRODUODOPA-R-foslevodopa-foscarbidopa-for-People-Living-with-Advanced-Parkinsons-Disease-in-the-European-Union. [Last accessed August, 2024].
81. de Andrade EM, Ghilardi MG, Cury RG, Barbosa ER, Fuentes R, Teixeira MJ, et al. Spinal cord stimulation for Parkinson's disease: a systematic review. Neurosurg Rev. 2016;39(1):27-35.
82. Liu X, Liu H, Liu Z, Rao J, Wang J, Wang P, et al. Transcranial Direct Current Stimulation for Parkinson's Disease: A Systematic Review and Meta-Analysis. Front Aging Neurosci. 2021;13: 746797.
83. Brinker D, Smilowska K, Paschen S, Antonini A, Moro E, Deuschl G. How to Use the New European Academy of Neurology/Movement Disorder Society European Section Guideline for Invasive Therapies in Parkinson's Disease. Mov Disord Clin Pract. 2024;11(3):209-19.
84. Schuepbach WMM, Rau J, Knudsen K, Volkmann J, Krack P, Timmermann L, et al. Neurostimulation for Parkinson's Disease with Early Motor Complications. N Engl J Med. 2013;368(7):610-22.

CHAPTER 4

Current Management of Dystonia

Manu SG, Asha Kishore

ABSTRACT

Dystonia is characterized by sustained or intermittent muscle contractions causing abnormal, often repetitive, movements, postures, or both. Treatment of dystonia is complicated due to the considerable heterogeneity in its etiology and clinical manifestations. A systematic clinical examination and diagnostic evaluation is necessary before appropriate treatment can be selected. Except in a small proportion of cases for which there is a specific etiology-based treatment, treatment of dystonia is mostly symptomatic, reflecting the deficits in our current understanding of the pathophysiological basis of most dystonias. The symptomatic treatment of dystonia includes oral medications, botulinum toxin (BT) therapy, and surgical interventions such as deep brain stimulation (DBS) or pallidotomy. Oral medications include drugs acting on various neurotransmitter systems, but generally clinical response is unsatisfactory. BT remains the mainstay therapy in patients with focal dystonia. The DBS is usually considered in severe cases of dystonia with significant functional impairment refractory to oral medications and/or BT therapy. This chapter mainly focuses on clinical indications and treatment principles of various available therapeutic options for dystonia.

Keywords: Dystonia, Treatment, Botulinum toxin for dystonia, DBS for dystonia.

INTRODUCTION

The definition and classification of dystonia have evolved over the last few decades with better understanding of the phenomenology and etiologies of dystonia. The current definition and classification scheme was proposed by a consensus group comprising an international panel of experts in 2013.[1] Accordingly, dystonia is defined as a movement disorder characterized by sustained or intermittent muscle contractions causing abnormal, often repetitive, movements, postures, or both. Dystonic movements are typically patterned, twisting, and may be tremulous. Dystonia is often initiated or worsened by voluntary action and may be associated with overflow of muscle activation. The current classification of dystonia is based on two axes: Axis I (Clinical features) and Axis II (Etiology).[1] Axis I describes the clinical phenomenology in a given patient based on five descriptors—age at onset (infancy, childhood, adolescence, early adulthood, and late adulthood), body distribution (focal, segmental, multifocal, generalized, and hemidystonia), temporal pattern, coexistence of other movement disorders (isolated and combined), and other neurological manifestations (complex). Axis II describes dystonia based on the identifiable anatomical changes and inheritance pattern. The anatomical changes can be characterized using neuroimaging or pathological examination and described as degenerative, structural or those without evidence for degenerative or structural lesions. Dystonia with a proven genetic cause is classified as inherited, whereas acquired group includes those with a specific, known, and acquired cause (perinatal brain injury, drug, infection, vascular, etc.).[1]

GENERAL ASPECTS OF TREATMENT OF DYSTONIA

Treatment of dystonia is mostly symptomatic except in a small proportion of cases for which there is a specific etiology-based treatment. This limitation reflects the deficits in our current understanding of the pathophysiological basis of most dystonias. The symptomatic treatment of dystonia includes oral medications, botulinum toxin (BT) therapy, and surgical interventions such as deep brain stimulation (DBS), or pallidotomy. The distribution of dystonia and its severity are the main factors determining the type of treatment. For adult onset—isolated, focal dystonia, and BT injection is the first-line treatment. In isolated and segmental dystonia, BT can be considered when only few muscle groups are involved. In adolescent and childhood-onset isolated, generalized dystonia with extensive and severe involvement, DBS may be required. Recently, genetics have evolved as an important predictor of treatment response to DBS in isolated generalized or segmental dystonia.

ORAL PHARMACOTHERAPY FOR MANAGEMENT OF DYSTONIA

Medical management of dystonia includes symptomatic or etiology-specific treatment. Etiology-specific treatment is available only for a small proportion of dystonia patients **(Table 1)**,[1-9] whereas symptomatic treatment remains the major strategy in the remaining patients. In combined and complex dystonia categories, coexisting manifestations such as parkinsonism, myoclonus, spasticity may require additional treatment.

TABLE 1: Diseases causing dystonia as a prominent clinical manifestation and having specific treatment.

Disease	Clinical features	Specific treatment
Dopa-responsive dystonia *(DYT-GCH1)*[2]	Childhood onset dystonia with diurnal fluctuation of symptoms, or late onset of parkinsonism	Levodopa
Parkinson's disease due to *Parkin* mutations[3]	Onset in young adulthood (mean age—32 years), lower limb dystonia, parkinsonism, and normal cognition	Marked and sustained response to levodopa, but associated with motor fluctuations and dyskinesia
Wilson disease[4]	Onset in young adulthood (range: 3–45 years of age). Children—usually presents with hepatic disease, less often with dystonia. In adults—neurological involvement can cause dystonia, parkinsonism, dysarthria, and psychiatric disturbances (depression, bipolar spectrum disorder, and psychosis)	Copper-chelating agents (D-penicillamine and trientine), and zinc

Continued

Continued

Disease	Clinical features	Specific treatment
PLA2G6-associated neurodegeneration (adult-onset dystonia-parkinsonism subtype)[5]	Onset in young adulthood age, neuropsychiatric manifestations (depression, personality changes, and delusions) followed by dystonia and parkinsonism	Levodopa—dramatic but short-lasting response, complicated by dyskinesia
Aceruloplasminemia[6]	Onset: 30–70 years of age; microcytic anemia, diabetes mellitus, retinal degeneration, neurological manifestations (dystonia, parkinsonism, ataxia, and cognitive impairment)	Iron-chelating agents—desferrioxamine, deferiprone (early iron chelation therapy can slow progression of neurological manifestations)
Niemann–Pick disease type C (adolescent and adulthood presentation)[7]	Onset—in adolescence or young adulthood; dystonia, ataxia, cognitive impairment, parkinsonism, and vertical supranuclear gaze palsy	Miglustat
Biotin-thiamine responsive basal ganglia disease (*SLC19A3* mutation)[8]	Classic presentation occurs in childhood (3–10 years) as recurrent episodes of confusion, seizures, dystonia, ataxia, rigidity, ophthalmoplegia, and dysphagia	Biotin and thiamine
Glutaric aciduria type 1[9]	Infantile onset of acute encephalopathic crisis (precipitated by fever, infections, vaccinations, etc.) causing acute bilateral striatal injury followed by (after 3 months to 3 years) complex movement disorders especially dystonia	Lysine restriction in diet and carnitine supplementation

SYMPTOMATIC TREATMENT OF DYSTONIA

For classification and understanding mechanism of action of various anti-dystonia medications we briefly discuss relevant neurochemistry of dystonia.[10-13] Striatum is composed of three cell types—striatal projection neurons (medium spiny neurons), matrix cells, and giant aspiny interneurons. Striatal projection neurons in rostral striatum gives origin to gamma-aminobutyric acid (GABA)-ergic striatonigral projections synapsing at substantia nigra pars compacta (SNc). Dopaminergic SNc neurons, in turn, project to matrix cells in dorsolateral putamen forming nigrostriatal pathway. Tonically, activated giant aspiny interneurons form cholinergic synapse with striosomes. Matrix neurons contain dopamine D1 and D2 receptors and innervate globus pallidus internus (GPi), globus pallidus externus (GPe), and substantia nigra reticulata (SNr), thereby influencing direct (via excitatory D1 receptors) and indirect pathways (via inhibitory D2 receptors) in basal ganglia.

Striosomes receive cholinergic innervation from striatal cholinergic interneurons and neurons in pedunculopontine nucleus. GABA is the main neurotransmitter of striosomes that synapses with pallidal neurons and SNc. Striosomes receive dopaminergic innervation from SNc via the nigrostriatal pathway. Drugs acting at these neurotransmitter systems at various levels have been found to be effective in dystonia. But, none of these drugs have been studied in any large scale, double-blinded, placebo-controlled trials and no oral medications have been approved by the Food and

Drug Administration (FDA) for treatment in dystonia. Evidence for these drugs is mostly based on small and controlled trials, retrospective studies, and anecdotal reports.

Drugs Acting on Cholinergic System

Hyperactivity of cholinergic interneurons in striatum has been implicated in dystonia. Anticholinergic drugs are the most commonly used pharmacological agent for dystonia. They act on the postsynaptic M1 receptors in striosomal neurons and are now used mostly in generalized dystonia.[14] Trihexyphenidyl is the most commonly used drug in this category followed by benztropine. A double-blind, placebo-controlled prospective cross-over randomized controlled trial (RCT) including 31 patients with idiopathic generalized or focal dystonia receiving trihexyphenidyl showed significant benefit in 71% patients, with 42% having sustained dramatic benefit at follow-up after 2.4 years.[15] One open label study including 35 patients with idiopathic generalized and focal dystonia showed significant symptomatic improvement in only 37% cases, whereas none of the nine patients with symptomatic dystonia showed adequate improvement.[16] Similar open-label studies showed improvement in 30–40% of patients with idiopathic generalized dystonia and a more variable rate of 12–50% among those with focal dystonia after treatment with trihexyphenidyl.[17,18] One double-blind and placebo-controlled RCT showed absence of clinical benefit with trihexyphenidyl in patients with dystonic cerebral palsy.[19] Thus, trihexyphenidyl can give clinical benefit only for a small proportion of patients with idiopathic generalized dystonia. Adverse effects of trihexyphenidyl include central side effects such as sedation, cognitive impairment, psychosis, chorea, and autonomic side effects such as mydriasis, dry mouth, urinary retention, and constipation. Sedation and memory impairment occur at relatively higher doses especially in elderly patients. Slow titration of the dose can reduce incidence of side effects and in case of central side effects dose reduction or drug withdrawal may be required. Children can usually tolerate higher doses compared to adults.[20]

Drugs Acting on GABAergic System

Baclofen

Baclofen is a GABA-B receptor agonist and is considered the next most effective agent for dystonia after anticholinergics. Though there are no placebo-controlled RCTs, retrospective studies and small case series showed clinical improvement in adult and pediatric patients.[21,22] Notably, some patients who show no response to anticholinergics may respond to baclofen.[21] Side effects include drowsiness, fatigue, nausea, giddiness. Abrupt withdrawal of baclofen can cause withdrawal syndrome characterized by dystonic storm, confusion, and seizures.

Intrathecal baclofen was tried in view of reduced cerebrospinal fluid (CSF) penetrance of oral baclofen and was found to be beneficial especially in patients with axial or lower limb predominant dystonia and coexisting spasticity.[23-25] Due to surgical procedure-related complications, hardware-related problems (infection and pump malfunction), and baclofen withdrawal syndrome, intrathecal baclofen is not a popular option currently.

Benzodiazepines

Benzodiazepines bind to GABA-A receptors and increase the frequency of chloride channel opening, thereby facilitating inhibitory signals. They are less effective than anticholinergics and are considered second- or third-line agents in dystonia.

There are no large and double-blind RCTs on use of benzodiazepines in dystonia. They are most useful in dystonia with prominent phasic components such as blepharospasm and dystonia with prominent tremors.[26,27] Clonazepam and diazepam are the preferred agents due to their longer half-life. Clonazepam may be particularly effective in myoclonus-dystonia syndrome.[28] Side effects include drowsiness, fatigue, ataxia, dizziness, behavioral abnormalities, and withdrawal syndrome.[29]

Drugs Acting on Dopaminergic System

These include: (1) Levodopa, and (2) Drugs reducing dopamine—presynaptic dopamine depletors (tetrabenazine) and postsynaptic dopamine-receptor blockers (clozapine and typical neuroleptics). Levodopa can be used in dopa-responsive dystonia (DRD) as an etiology-specific agent or as a symptomatic drug in other forms of dystonia. Due to its dramatic response in DRD, levodopa trial should be given to all patients with suggestive phenotype. In children and young adults with focal or generalized dystonia, if DRD cannot be excluded, a trial of levodopa is warranted. Some patients may respond to doses as low as 100/25 mg/day of levodopa/carbidopa, but administration of 1,000 mg/day of levodopa for 1 month is required for adequate assessment of treatment response.[2,30] Mechanism of action of levodopa in other forms of dystonia is not clearly understood.

Tetrabenazine is a vesicular monoamine transporter 2 (VMAT2) inhibitor and prevents vesicular reuptake of dopamine in presynaptic nerve terminal, thereby reducing the level of dopamine in synaptic cleft. It is not usually used as a first-line agent in dystonia but used as a common drug in tardive dystonia.[31] Common side effects of tetrabenazine include sedation, depression, and parkinsonism. Recently, few placebo-controlled RCTs showed that new VMAT2 inhibitors, deutetrabenazine, and valbenazine have good clinical benefits in tardive dystonia with fewer side effects.[32,33]

Dopamine-receptor blockers can cause acute dystonic reactions and tardive syndromes including tardive dystonia, but paradoxically they can be useful in the treatment of dystonia. Though these drugs were used for management of dystonia in the past, currently they are not popular due to the propensity to cause tardive syndromes.[34] Risk for causing tardive syndrome is related to D2 blocking potential of these agents and hence clozapine (with higher affinity for D4 receptors) can be used for treatment of dystonia. Blood counts should be monitored due to the risk for agranulocytosis while patient is on clozapine.[35]

In general, drugs reducing dopamine levels are used in tardive dystonia or in generalized dystonia when other medications are ineffective. Tetrabenazine is the preferred drug in this category followed by clozapine.[36]

Other Medications

Some medications have been shown to have modest effect in treatment of dystonia. These include sodium oxybate, zolpidem, and cannabinoids.[37-39] Sodium oxybate may be particularly effective in myoclonus-dystonia syndrome.[28] Zonisamide, which is an anticonvulsant, that blocks voltage-dependent sodium and calcium channels have also been found to be effective in myoclonus-dystonia in a double-blind crossover trial.[40] Due to unproven therapeutic efficacy, these medications are not used in routine clinical practice for management of dystonia **(Table 2)**.

TABLE 2: Dosage and side effects of common symptomatic antidystonia medications.[36]

Drug	Initial starting dose	Titration*	Usual therapeutic daily dose	Maximum dose in dystonia	Side effects
Trihexyphenidyl	2 mg/day; in three divided doses	2–3 mg/day	15 mg/day (in childhood generalized dystonia)	120 mg/day (in childhood generalized dystonia)	Sedation, cognitive impairment, psychosis, dry mouth, urinary retention, and constipation
Baclofen	10 mg/day; in three divided doses	10–15 mg/day	30 mg/day	120 mg/day	Drowsiness, fatigue, dizziness, and nausea
Clonazepam	0.25 mg/day; in two divided doses	0.25 mg/day	1 mg/day	6 mg/day	Sedation, depression, and behavioral changes
Tetrabenazine	12.5 mg/day; in three divided doses	12.5 mg/day	37.5 mg/day	200 mg/day	Drowsiness, depression, and parkinsonism

*Titration to be done slowly; once in every 3–4 days in children and young adults; once in every week in older adults and patients prone to side effects.

GENERAL PRINCIPLES IN SYMPTOMATIC MEDICAL MANAGEMENT OF DYSTONIA

In general, one of the drugs is started at the lowest dose and titrated up slowly until therapeutic effect is attained or dose-limiting side effects appear. In case of adverse effects, the dose needs to be reduced until these resolve, or the drug may have to be stopped if side effects persist. If adequate clinical improvement cannot be attained with relatively high dose of a drug, then a second medication can be added. There are no RCTs comparing various antidystonia medications to give recommendations on selection of the initial drug. Usually, trihexyphenidyl is used as the initial agent, with baclofen and clonazepam used as the second-line medication. A trial of levodopa (for at least 3 months up to a dose of 600 mg/day or 10 mg/kg/day) has to be given in children and young patients with dystonia if the presentation resembles DRD.[41] Zonisamide, clonazepam, and sodium oxybate may be preferred in myoclonus-dystonia syndrome. In tardive dystonia, tetrabenazine and clozapine are used as first-line agents.

BOTULINUM TOXIN INJECTION FOR DYSTONIA

Dystonia is one of the most important indications for use of BT. Botulinum toxin can be combined with oral medications, DBS, and physiotherapy for optimal outcomes in the management of dystonia.[42]

Botulinum toxin drug is a complex mixture comprising BT and excipients. BT component includes botulinum neurotoxin (BNT) and complexing proteins. BNT can be of seven different serotypes (BNT types A, B, C, D, E, F, and G), among which BNT types A and B are approved for clinical use by the FDA. Excipients include substances for stabilization and pH calibration of the BT drug.[43]

Botulinum toxin can impair cholinergic neurotransmission at neuromuscular junction and cholinergic autonomic innervation of salivary, lacrimal, and sweat glands. When BT is injected into target muscle, it reaches the cholinergic nerve terminal and binds to glycoprotein structures with high affinity. Then, it gets internalized and cleaves various proteins (SNARE proteins) involved in acetyl choline transport from nerve terminal to synaptic cleft. BNT serotype A, C, and E target SNAP-25, whereas serotypes B, D, and F target VAMP protein.[44] This difference in affinity explains varying therapeutic efficacy among different BT drugs. This interruption of synaptic transmission by BT is only temporary with eventual regeneration of synapses.[45] Clinically, this effect translates as peripheral paresis which is localized, well controllable, and follows a distinct and predictable time course. Clinical effects of BT start 2–3 days after injection, peak at around 2 weeks, plateau, and start declining after 2–3 months.

Botulinum toxin formulations approved by the FDA include onabotulinumtoxinA (ONA, Botox, Allergan Inc., Irvine, CA, USA), abobotulinumtoxinA (ABO, Dysport®, Ipsen Ltd., Slough, Berks., UK), incobotulinumtoxinA (INCO, Xeomin, Merz Pharmaceuticals, Frankfurt/M, Germany) and rimabotulinumtoxinB (RIMA, NeuroBloc/Myobloc, Solstice Neurosciences Inc., Malvern, PA, USA).[46,47] ONA, ABO, and INCO are based on BNT type A whereas RIMA contains BNT serotype B. All BT-A drugs are available in powder form, which is reconstituted with normal saline or sterile water prior to use. Usually 100 MU of ONA/INCO is diluted in 2.5 mL of normal saline or sterile water before injection.[48] BT has very long shelf-life prior to reconstitution, but once reconstituted, it has to be used within 24 hours. Special storage temperatures are required for all BT preparations except INCO which can be stored at room temperature.[43] The biological activity of therapeutic BT preparations is expressed in mouse unit (MU). One mouse unit is the amount of BT which would kill 50% of a BT-intoxicated mouse population. Activity assays used by the manufacturers are performed differently so that the activity labeling of the different BT drugs cannot be compared directly. One mouse unit of ONA is equivalent to approximately 2.5 MU of ABO, 1 MU of INCO, and 50 MU of RIMA.[47]

Adverse effects related to BT are usually caused by local diffusion to adjacent tissues and its severity and duration depend on the dose as well as the injection technique. Side effects usually start 1 week after injection and last for 1–2 weeks.[48] BNT-B type is associated with relatively more autonomic side effects like dryness of mouth, difficulties with accommodation of eyes, etc.[47] Other side effects include hypersensitivity reactions, injection site infections, and injection site bleeding or bruising. Long-term use of BT can result in development of immunogenicity due to the formation of neutralizing antibodies which can result in therapeutic failure.[49] Immunogenicity varies with BNT serotype and is reported to be as low as 0% for INCO and as high as 42.4% for RIMA.[50] Short inter-dose interval between BT injections and higher cumulative dose of BT are other factors associated with higher risk for immunogenicity.[51]

General Principles of Botulinum Toxin Therapy in Dystonia

The basic principle of BT therapy in dystonia is to select appropriate target muscles and to choose the appropriate BT dose for each of the selected muscles. The target muscles are selected based on clinical examination and the pathological position or movements of the involved body part. Clinical examination involves palpation of the involved muscles after active contraction and application of the knowledge of anatomical surface landmarks. EMG or ultrasound may be used to guide injection.[52] The dose of BT is decided such that it is as low as possible to avoid any functional impairment, but high enough to produce optimal therapeutic effect.[42,48,53] Each muscle has a therapeutic window for BT injection identified from previous studies, which is modified by several factors. Higher therapeutic range can be used if pathological muscle activity is strong and agonist muscles performing similar action are available. Lower limits are preferred when pathological activity is functionally useful. Factors related to reduced muscle mass (old age, female sex, and atrophy related to previous BT use) necessitates lower BT dose, whereas higher doses are required in patients with athletic physique.[53] The maximum total dose of BT in a single session was previously recommended was 300–400 MU of INCO, but recent studies have established the safety of dosages up to 1,250 MU of INCO (High-dose of BT therapy).[54] Subsequent doses can be decided based on treatment efficacy and presence of side effects with the initial dose. In case of suboptimal therapeutic effect with the first injection, subsequent dose for that muscle can be increased or if side effects appeared in the initial session, the dose can be reduced in later sessions. When therapeutic response is persistently low despite the higher dose of BT, muscle selection has to be reconsidered. The previously recommended inter-dose interval of 12 weeks was challenged in recent studies which established the safety of BT injection in as short as 6-week intervals (short interval of BT therapy).[55]

BOTULINUM TOXIN IN CERVICAL DYSTONIA

The clinical spectrum of abnormal head and neck posture in cervical dystonia (CD) is extremely heterogenous due to the variable degrees of involvement of the muscles maintaining head and neck posture. BT injection into the involved muscles is the preferred treatment for CD and it has a response rate of around 80% in several open labeled and double-blind studies.[56] Among the 54 muscles involved in maintaining head and neck posture, only a few large neck muscles usually contribute to the dystonic posture, and these are selected for BT injection.[48]

According to the recently introduced Col-Cap concept, head and neck movement can occur functionally at two different levels with C2 vertebrae as a fixed point. In the upper level, movement occurs between head and C2, whereas in the lower level this occurs between C2 and C7. When muscles rostral to C3 are involved in dystonia, head can rotate or tilt in relation to neck with C2 vertebrae as fulcrum producing rotational torticaput or laterocaput, respectively. Similarly, involvement of muscles caudal to C3 vertebrae can cause neck movement in relation to trunk producing rotational torticollis or laterocollis. Larynx can serve as a useful surface landmark for differentiating these two, which gets displaced laterally in collis but remains in midline in caput. Anterocollis/retrocollis and anterocaput/retrocaput can be similarly differentiated[48,57] **(Tables 3 and 4)**.

Common side effects include dysphagia and neck weakness. These are usually transient and last for 1 or 2 weeks.

BOTULINUM TOXIN IN OROMANDIBULAR DYSTONIA

Oromandibular dystonia (OMD) is a type of focal dystonia involving muscles of mastication, lower facial, labial and lingual muscles. OMD with involvement of muscles of mastication can cause jaw opening dystonia, jaw closing dystonia, lateral deviation, protrusion, and retraction or a combination of any of these **(Tables 5 and 6)**.

TABLE 3: Types of cervical dystonia (CD) and muscles involved.[48,57]

Type of cervical dystonia	Muscles commonly used for BT injection
Rotational collis (Torticollis)	• Contralateral sternocleidomastoid • Contralateral trapezius • Ipsilateral splenius capitis • Ipsilateral levator scapulae
Laterocollis	• Ipsilateral sternocleidomastoid • Ipsilateral trapezius • Ipsilateral levator scapulae • Ipsilateral splenius capitis
Anterocollis	• Bilateral sternocleidomastoid • Bilateral scalenus • Bilateral longus colli
Retrocollis	• Bilateral splenius capitis and cervicis • Bilateral semispinalis capitis and cervicis
Rotational caput (Torticaput)	• Contralateral sternocleidomastoid • Contralateral trapezius • Ipsilateral obliquus capitis inferior
Laterocaput	• Ipsilateral sternocleidomastoid • Ipsilateral trapezius • Ipsilateral splenius capitis
Anterocaput	• Bilateral levator scapulae • Bilateral longus capitis • Bilateral sternocleidomastoid
Retrocaput	• Bilateral trapezius • Bilateral obliquus capitis inferior • Bilateral semispinalis capitis

TABLE 4: Typical dose of BT (ONA and INCO, in MU) used in CD.[53]

Target muscle	Typical dose (mean dose) (in MU)	Dose variability (standard deviation)	Dose range (minimum–maximum)
Trapezius (Pars descendens)	44.7	27.5	10–200
Trapezius (Pars horizontalis)	46.0	27.4	20–180
Splenius capitis	55.2	33.2	10–300
Sternocleidomastoid	46.4	21.1	10–120
Levator scapulae	34.2	15.3	10–80
Deep neck muscles	32.2	15.4	20–60

(BT: botulinum toxin; CD: cervical dystonia; INCO: incobotulinumtoxinA; MU: mouse units; ONA: onabotulinumtoxinA)

TABLE 5: Types of oromandibular dystonia (OMD) and muscles involved.[48]

Types of OMD	Muscles usually selected for BT injection
Jaw-closing OMD	Massetter—initial muscle used for denervation. If response is inadequate—Temporalis and medial pterygoid can be injected
Jaw-opening OMD	Lateral pterygoid
Jaw-deviating OMD	• Contralateral lateral pterygoid • Ipsilateral medial pterygoid • Ipsilateral temporalis

TABLE 6: Typical dose of BT (ONA and INCO, in MU) used in OMD.[53]

Target muscle	Typical dose (mean dose) (in MU)	Dose variability (standard deviation)	Dose range (minimum–maximum)
Massetter	36.7	14	20–60
Pterygoid	31.6	13.2	8–60
Temporalis	42.0	23.9	20–80

(BT: botulinum toxin; INCO: incobotulinumtoxinA; MU: mouse units; OMA: oromandibular dystonia; ONA: onabotulinumtoxinA)

BOTULINUM TOXIN IN WRITER'S CRAMP

Dystonic contractions can occur while doing particular action and can be specific for a particular task. Writer's cramp is a focal task specific hand dystonia. Simple writer's cramp involves difficulty only in writing, whereas complex writer's cramp or dystonic writer's cramp refers to those who have dystonia in other tasks besides writing.[48,58]

Botulinum toxin injection is the most promising treatment available for writer's cramp, and its efficacy depends on accurate identification of involved muscle. Muscles involved in writer's cramp can be identified by careful clinical examination of patient at rest and during writing. The patient should be asked to write without trying to compensate and should describe any pulling sensation in forearm or hand muscles while writing. Writing with nondominant hand can elicit dystonia in dominant hand (mirror dystonia) and this can be used to identify dystonic muscles and differentiate dystonia from compensatory muscle activity. EMG guidance is recommended especially for targeting deeper muscles **(Tables 7 and 8)**.[48]

DEEP BRAIN STIMULATION IN DYSTONIA

Deep brain stimulation has been proved in randomized double-blind sham-controlled studies to be effective treatment for patients with drug refractory dystonia causing significant functional impairment.[59,60] In DBS, controlled direct current from an implantable pulse generator is used for stimulation of a specific subcortical nucleus through electrodes. GPi, ventralis intermediate (VIM) nucleus of thalamus, and subthalamic nucleus (STN) have been studied as DBS targets in dystonia. The typical DBS target for dystonia is GPi, but recent studies showed comparable effects with STN DBS.[61]

A recent systematic review compared the outcomes among dystonia patients who underwent DBS in GPi versus STN (35 studies, including 319 GPi DBS and 113 STN DBS patients).[62] Both GPi and STN DBS were found to be associated with significant improvement

TABLE 7: Types of writer's cramp and muscles involved.[48]

Subtype of Writer's cramp	Muscles involved
Focal flexor (finger) subtype	• Flexor pollicis longus • Flexor pollicis brevis
Generalized flexor (wrist) subtype with/without finger flexion	• Flexor carpi radialis • Flexor carpi ulnaris • Flexor digitorum superficialis • Flexor digitorum profundus • Palmaris longus • Pronator teres • Pronator quadratus
Focal extensor (finger) subtype	• Extensor pollicis longus • Extensor indicis proprius
Generalized extensor subtype	• Extensor carpi radialis longus • Extensor carpi radialis brevis • Extensor carpi ulnaris • Extensor digitorum communis • Extensor indicis proprius • Extensor pollicis longus • Extensor pollicis brevis • Abductor pollicis longus

TABLE 8: Typical dose of BT used in Writer's cramp.[53]

Target muscle	Typical dose (mean dose) (in MU)	Dose variability (standard deviation)	Dose range (minimum–maximum)
Flexor pollicis longus	22.7	13.5	6–60
Flexor carpi ulnaris	32.7	18.2	10–80
Flexor carpi radialis	13.0	5.5	8–20
Flexor digitorum superficialis	21.8	13.9	8–70
Flexor digitorum profundus	19.9	10.3	8–40
Pronator teres	47.0	39.3	8–100
Extensor pollicis	9.3	1.2	8–10
Extensor indicis	34.3	43.8	10–100
Extensor carpi ulnaris	35.4	13.1	10–60
Extensor carpi radialis	28.0	13.2	10–50

(BT: botulinum toxin; MU: mouse units)

in movement symptoms as well as quality of life. As far as body distribution of dystonia is considered, this systematic review reported significant improvement in patients with focal, segmental, and generalized dystonia. CD was reported to show dramatic response after DBS in several studies.[63] Considering the etiology of dystonia, primary (idiopathic or isolated genetic dystonia), secondary hereditary [e.g., pantothenate kinase-associated neurodegeneration (PKAN) and Wilson disease] and secondary nonhereditary (acquired) dystonia patients were found to show significant improvement after DBS. The improvement was the highest among patients with primary dystonia followed by secondary nonhereditary group and was least for secondary hereditary dystonia.[62] A meta-analysis of DBS in dyskinetic cerebral palsy (including 20 articles, 68 patients) showed only modest benefit in movement symptoms and quality of life.[62,64] Patients with tardive dystonia showed good benefit comparable to that in isolated or idiopathic dystonia.[65-67] Genetics plays an important role in determining DBS outcome in dystonia patients. *DYT-TOR1A* has been shown to have the most significant clinical outcome after DBS in comparison to other monogenic forms of dystonia.[68] Treatment response is less favorable in *DYT-THAP1* cases with a variable improvement ranging from 16 to 72%.[69] *DYT-ANO3* is associated with tremor-dominant CD, and hence VIM-DBS may be more beneficial.[70-72] Previous studies showed that GPi DBS offers significant benefit in *DYT-SGCE* (myoclonus-dystonia syndrome).[73] VIM-DBS has also been reported to be effective for dystonic tremor and myoclonus in *DYT-SGCE* and can be used along with GPi-DBS.[74] A recent systematic review reported effectiveness of pallidal stimulation in *KMT2B*-associated dystonia.[75] Small case series showed good response in patients with *DYT-GNAL* after GPi-DBS.[76-81] Thus, genetic testing in dystonia patients before DBS procedure can help to predict the outcome prediction and counsel patients and families accordingly. Adverse effects were less among patients with primary dystonia compared to secondary hereditary and secondary nonhereditary dystonia.[62] Though there were no prognostic factors identified in the meta-analysis, other studies showed that younger age at DBS and shorter duration of symptoms were associated with better prognosis while caudate atrophy in MRI was associated with poor prognosis after DBS.[13-16]

Overall, patients with idiopathic or inherited, isolated, focal, segmental, or generalized dystonia, tardive dystonia and myoclonus-dystonia respond well to DBS. Acquired dystonia secondary to brain injuries and neurodegenerative disorders typically respond less well. Among patients with favorable prognostic features, factors that negatively affect the outcome including secondary skeletal deformities, secondary disabilities such as myelopathy, age, disease duration, and genetic subtype need to be considered before proceeding with DBS.

CONCLUSION

The treatment of dystonia is complicated due to the considerable heterogeneity in etiology and clinical manifestations. A systematic clinical examination and diagnostic evaluation is necessary before appropriate treatment can be selected. DBS has proven to be an effective treatment in selected situations and many patients get meaningful symptomatic benefit with it. However, the knowledge gap in this field is still high and carries a lot of scope for newer therapeutic strategies. Development of new BT preparations with higher therapeutic efficacy and lesser immunogenicity, identification of predictors of response to DBS can refine existing treatment strategies in dystonia. Improvement in our knowledge of pathophysiology of dystonia might result in the development of new pharmacological agents or therapeutic interventions in future. With the advancement in genetic diagnostic technologies, targeted therapies might be available in future for specific types of dystonia.

REFERENCES

1. Albanese A, Bhatia K, Bressman SB, Delong MR, Fahn S, Fung VS, et al. Phenomenology and classification of dystonia: a consensus update. Mov Disord. 2013;28(7):863-73.
2. Kim R, Jeon B, Lee WW. A Systematic Review of Treatment Outcome in Patients with Dopa-responsive Dystonia (DRD) and DRD-Plus. Mov Disord Clin Pract. 2016;3:435-42.
3. Lücking CB, Dürr A, Bonifati V, Vaughan J, Michele GD, Gasser T, et al. Association between Early-Onset Parkinson's Disease and Mutations in the Parkin Gene. N Engl J Med. 2000;342:1560-7.
4. Rodriguez-Castro KI, Hevia-Urrutia FJ, Sturniolo GC. Wilson's disease: A review of what we have learned. World J Hepatol. 2015;7(29):2859-70.
5. Gregory A, Kurian MA, Maher ER, Hogarth P, Hayflick SJ. PLA2G6-Associated Neurodegeneration. In: Adam MP, Feldman J, Mirzaa GM, et al. (Eds). GeneReviews®. Seattle (WA): University of Washington; 1993-2014.
6. Giacomo M, Fabiana B, Acaynne LZ, Annalisa C, Domenico G. Aceruloplasminemia: A Severe Neurodegenerative Disorder Deserving an Early Diagnosis. Front Neurosci. 2009;13:325.
7. Lad M, Thomas RH, Anderson K, Griffiths TD. Niemann-Pick type C: contemporary diagnosis and treatment of a classical disorder. Pract Neurol. 2019;19:420-3.
8. Algahtani H, Ghamdi S, Shirah B, Alharbi B, Algahtani R, Bazaid A. Biotin–thiamine–responsive basal ganglia disease: catastrophic consequences of delay in diagnosis and treatment. Neurol Res. 2016;39(2):117-25.
9. Larson A, Goodman S. Glutaric Acidemia Type 1. In: Adam MP, Feldman J, Mirzaa GM, et al. (eds). GeneReviews® [Internet]. Seattle (WA): University of Washington, Seattle; 1993-2024.
10. Crittenden JR, Graybiel AM. Basal Ganglia disorders associated with imbalances in the striatal striosome and matrix compartments. Front Neuroanat. 2011;5:59.
11. Matsushima A, Graybiel AM. Combinatorial developmental controls on striatonigral circuits. Cell Rep. 2020;31(11):107778.
12. Sato K, Sumi-Ichinose C, Kaji R, Ikemoto K, Nomura T, Nagatsu I, et al. Differential involvement of striosome and matrix dopamine systems in a transgenic model of dopa-responsive dystonia. Proc Natl Acad Sci USA. 2008;105(34):12551-6.
13. Brüggemann N. Contemporary functional neuroanatomy and pathophysiology of dystonia. J Neural Transm. 2021;128:499-508.
14. Jankovic J. Treatment of dystonia. Lancet Neurol. 2006;5:864-72.
15. Burke RE, Fahn S, Marsden CD. Torsion dystonia: a double-blind, prospective trial of high-dosage trihexyphenidyl. Neurology. 1986;36:160-4.
16. Lang AE. High dose anticholinergic therapy in adult dystonia. Can J Neurol Sci. 1986;13(1):42-6.
17. Fahn S. High dosage anticholinergic therapy in dystonia. Neurology (Cleveland). 1983;33:1255-61.
18. Marsden CD, Marion MH, Quinn N. The treatment of severe dystonia in children and adults. J Neurol Neurosurg Psychiatry. 1984;47:1166-73.
19. Harvey AR, Baker LB, Reddihough DS, Scheinberg A, Williams K. Trihexyphenidyl for dystonia in cerebral palsy. Cochrane Database Syst Rev. 2018;5(5):CD012430.
20. Jankovic J. Medical treatment of dystonia. Mov Disord. 2013;28:1001-12.
21. Greene P, Shale H, Fahn S. Analysis of open-label trials in torsion dystonia using high dosages of anticholinergics and other drugs. Mov Disord. 1988;3:46-60.
22. Greene PE, Fahn S. Baclofen in the treatment of idiopathic dystonia in children. Mov Disord. 1992;7:48-52.
23. Narayan RK, Loubser PG, Jankovic J, Donovan WH, Bontke CF. Intrathecal baclofen for intractable axial dystonia. Neurology. 1991;41:1141-2.
24. Butler C, Campbell S. Evidence of the effects of intrathecal baclofen for spastic and dystonic cerebral palsy. AACPDM Treatment Outcomes Committee Review Panel. Dev Med Child Neurol. 2000;42:634-45.
25. Albright AL, Barry MJ, Painter MJ, Shultz B. Infusion of intrathecal baclofen for generalized dystonia in cerebral palsy. J Neurosurg. 1998;88:73-6.
26. Fasano A, Bove F, Lang AE. The treatment of dystonic tremor: a systematic review. J Neurol Neurosurg Psychiatry. 2014;85:759-69.
27. Jankovic J, Ford J. Blepharospasm and orofacial-cervical dystonia: clinical and pharmacological findings in 100 patients. Ann Neurol. 1983;13:402-11.
28. Fearon C, Peall KJ, Vidailhet M, Fasano A. Medical management of myoclonus-dystonia and implications for underlying pathophysiology. Parkinsonism Relat Disord. 2020;77:48-56.
29. Greene P, Shale H, Fahn S. Experience with high dosages of anticholinergic and other drugs in the treatment of torsion dystonia. Adv Neurol. 1988;50:547-56.

30. Weissbach A, Pauly MG, Herzog R, Hahn L, Halmans S, Hamami F, et al. Relationship of Genotype, Phenotype, and Treatment in Dopa-Responsive Dystonia: MDSGene Review. Mov Disord. 2022;37:0237-52.
31. Jankovic J, Clarence-Smith K. Tetrabenazine for the treatment of chorea and other hyperkinetic movement disorders. Expert Rev Neurother. 2011;11:1509-23.
32. Fernandez HH, Factor SA, Hauser RA, Jimenez-Shahed J, Ondo WG, Jarskog LF, et al. Randomized controlled trial of deutetrabenazine for tardive dyskinesia: The ARM-TD study. Neurology. 2017;88(21):2003-10.
33. Kane JM, Correll CU, Liang GS, Burke J, O'Brien CF. Efficacy of Valbenazine (NBI-98854) in Treating Subjects with Tardive Dyskinesia and Schizophrenia or Schizoaffective Disorder. Psychopharmacol Bull. 2017;47(3):69-76.
34. Jankovic J. Treatment of hyperkinetic movement disorders. Lancet Neurol. 2009;8:844-56.
35. Karp BI, Goldstein SR, Chen R, Samii A, Bara-Jimenez W, Hallett M. An open trial of clozapine for dystonia. Mov Disord. 1999;14:652-7.
36. Termsarasab P, Thammongkolchai T, Frucht SJ. Medical treatment of dystonia. J Clin Mov Disord. 2016;3:19. Erratum in: J Clin Mov Disord. 2018;5:8.
37. Simonyan K, Frucht SJ, Blitzer A, Sichani AH, Rumbach AF. A novel therapeutic agent, sodium oxybate, improves dystonic symptoms via reduced network-wide activity. Sci Rep. 2018;8(1):16111.
38. Miyazaki Y, Sako W, Asanuma K, Izumi Y, Miki T, Kaji R. Efficacy of zolpidem for dystonia: a study among different subtypes. Front Neurol. 2012;3:58.
39. Koppel BS. Cannabis in the Treatment of Dystonia, Dyskinesias, and Tics. Neurotherapeutics. 2015;12:788-92.
40. Hainque E, Vidailhet M, Cozic N, Charbonnier-Beaupel F, Thobois S, Tranchant C, et al. A randomized, controlled, double-blind, crossover trial of zonisamide in myoclonus-dystonia. Neurology. 2016;86(18):1729-35.
41. Malek N, Fletcher N, Newman E. Diagnosing Dopamine-Responsive Dystonias. Pract Neurol. 2015;15:340-5.
42. Dressler D, Adib Saberi F, Rosales RL. Botulinum toxin therapy of dystonia. J Neural Transm (Vienna). 2021;128(4):531-7.
43. Huang W, Foster JA, Rogachefsky AS. Pharmacology of botulinum toxin. J Am Acad Dermatol. 2000;43(2):249-59.
44. Blasi J, Chapman ER, Link E, Binz T, Yamasaki S, De Camilli P, et al. Botulinum neurotoxin: A selectively cleaves the synaptic protein SNAP-25. Nature. 1993;365:160-3.
45. de Paiva A, Meunier FA, Molgo J, Aoki KR, Dolly JO. Functional repair of motor endplates after botulinum neurotoxin type A poisoning: Biphasic switch of synaptic activity between nerve sprouts and their parent terminals. Proc Natl Acad Sci USA. 1999;96:3200-5.
46. Camargo CHF, Teive HAG. Use of botulinum toxin for movement disorders. Drugs Context. 2019:8: 1-14.
47. Jankovic J. Botulinum toxin: State of the art. Mov Disord. 2017;32:1131-8.
48. Truong D, Dressler D, Hallett M, Zachary C. Manual of Botulinum Toxin Therapy, 2nd edition. Cambridge: Cambridge University Press; 2014.
49. Albrecht P, Jansen A, Lee JI, Moll M, Ringelstein M, Rosenthal D, et al. High prevalence of neutralizing antibodies after long-term botulinum neurotoxin therapy. Neurology. 2019;92:E48-E54.
50. Bellows S, Jankovic J. Immunogenicity associated with botulinum toxin treatment. Toxins. 2019;11: 491.
51. Jankovic J, Schwartz K. Response and immuno-resistance to botulinum toxin injections. Neurology. 1995;45:1743-6.
52. Dressler D. Electromyographic evaluation of cervical dystonia for planning of botulinum toxin therapy. Eur J Neurol. 2000;7:713-8.
53. Dressler D, Altavista MC, Altenmueller E, Bhidayasiri R, Bohlega S, Chana P, et al. Consensus guidelines for botulinum toxin therapy: general algorithms and dosing tables for dystonia and spasticity. J Neural Transm (Vienna). 2021;128(3):321-35.
54. Dressler D, Adib Saberi F, Kollewe K, Schrader C. Safety aspects of IncobotulinumtoxinA high dose therapy. J Neural Transm. 2014a;122:327-33.
55. Dressler D, Adib Saberi F. Immunological safety of incobotulinumtoxinA (Xeomin®) therapy with reduced interinjection intervals. J Neural Transm. 2017;124:437-40.
56. Wissel J, Kanovsky P, Ruzicka E, Bares M, Hortova H, Streitova H, et al. Efficacy and safety of a standardised 500 unit dose of Dysport (clostridium botulinum toxin type A haemaglutinin complex) in a heterogeneous cervical dystonia population: results of a prospective, multicentre, randomised, double-blind, placebo-controlled, parallel group study. J Neurol. 2001;248(12):1073-8.
57. Jost WH, Tatu L. Selection of Muscles for Botulinum Toxin Injections in Cervical Dystonia. Mov Disord Clin Pract. 2015;2(3):224-6.

58. Marsden CD, Sheehy MP. Writer's cramp. Trends Neurosci. 1990;13(4):148-53.
59. Kupsch A, Benecke R, Müller J, Trottenberg T, Schneider GH, Poewe W, et al. Pallidal deep-brain stimulation in primary generalized or segmental dystonia. N Engl J Med. 2006;355(19):1978.
60. Volkmann J, Mueller J, Deuschl G, Kuhn AA, Krauss JK, Poewe W, et al.; the DBS study group for dystonia. Pallidal neurostimulation in patients with medication-refractory cervical dystonia: a randomised, sham-controlled trial. Lancet Neurology. 2014;13(9):875-84.
61. Cury RG, Kalia SK, Shah BB, Jimenez-Shahed J, Prashanth LK, Moro E. Surgical treatment of dystonia. Expert Rev Neurother. 2018.
62. Fan H, Zheng Z, Yin Z, Zhang J, Lu G. Deep Brain Atimulation Treating Dystonia: A Systematic Review of Targets, Body Distributions and Etiology Classifications. Front Hum Neurosci. 2021;15:757579.
63. Ostrem JL, Marks WJ Jr, Volz MM, Heath SL, Starr PA. Pallidal deep brain stimulation in patients with cranial-cervical dystonia (Meige syndrome). Mov Disord. 2007;22:1885-91.
64. Koy A, Hellmich M, Pauls KA, Marks W, Lin JP, Fricke O, et al. Effects of deep brain stimulation in dyskinetic cerebral palsy: a meta-analysis. Mov Disord. 2013;28:647-54.
65. Trottenberg T, Volkmann J, Deuschl G, Kühn AA, Schneider GH, Müller J, et al. Treatment of severe tardive dystonia with pallidal deep brain stimulation. Neurology. 2005;64:344-6.
66. Sako W, Goto S, Shimazu H, Murase N, Matsuzaki K, Tamura T, et al. Bilateral deep brain stimulation of the globus pallidus internus in tardive dystonia. Mov Disord. 2008;23:1929-31.
67. Shaikh AG, Mewes K, DeLong MR, Gross RE, Triche SD, Jinnah HA, et al. Temporal profile of improvement of tardive dystonia after globus pallidus deep brain stimulation. Parkinsonism Relat Disord. 2015;21:116-9.
68. Artusi CA, Dwivedi A, Romagnolo A, Bortolani S, Marsili L, Imbalzano G, et al. Differential response to pallidal deep brain stimulation among monogenic dystonias: systematic review and meta-analysis. J Neurol Neurosurg Psychiatry. 2020;91:426-33.
69. Tisch S, Kumar KR. Pallidal deep brain stimulation for monogenic dystonia: the effect of gene on outcome. Front Neurol. 2021;11:630391.
70. Moro E, LeReun C, Krauss JK, Albanese A, Lin JP, Walleser Autiero S, et al. Efficacy of pallidal stimulation in isolated dystonia: a systematic review and meta-analysis. Eur J Neurol. 2017;24:552-60.
71. Andrews C, Aviles-Olmos I, Hariz M, Foltynie T. Which patients with dystonia benefit from deep brain stimulation? A metaregression of individual patient outcomes. J Neurol Neurosurg Psychiatry. 2010;81:1383-89.
72. Jinnah HA, Alterman R, Klein C, Krauss JK, Moro E, Vidailhet M, et al. Deep brain stimulation for dystonia: a novel perspective on the value of genetic testing. J Neural Transm Vienna Austria 1996. 2017;124:417-30.
73. Wang X, Yu X. Deep brain stimulation for myoclonus dystonia syndrome: a meta-analysis with individual patient data. Neurosurg Rev. 2021;44:451-62.
74. Trottenberg T, Meissner W, Arnold G, Einhaupl KM, Kupsch A, Kabus C, et al. Neurostimulation of the ventral intermediate thalamic nucleus in inherited myoclonus-dystonia syndrome. Mov Disord. 2001;16:769-71.
75. Rajan R, Garg K, Saini A, Radhakrishnan DM, Carecchio M, Bk B, et al. GPi-DBS for KMT2B-Associated Dystonia: Systematic Review and Meta-Analysis. Mov Disord Clin Pract. 2021;9(1):31-7.
76. Sarva H, Trosch R, Kiss ZHT, Furtado S, Luciano MS, Glickman A, et al. Deep Brain Stimulation in Isolated Dystonia With a GNAL Mutation. Mov Disord. 2019;34(2):301-3.
77. Ahn JH, Kim AR, Kim NKD, Park WY, Kim JS, Kim M, et al. The Effect of Globus Pallidus Interna Deep Brain Stimulation on a Dystonia Patient with the GNAL Mutation Compared to Patients with DYT1 and DYT6. J Mov Disord. 2019;12(2):120-4.
78. Eltahawy HA, Saint-Cyr J, Giladi N, Lang AE, Lozano AM. Primary dystonia is more responsive than secondary dystonia to pallidal interventions: outcome after pallidotomy or pallidal deep brain stimulation. Neurosurgery. 2004;54:613-9; discussion 619-21.
79. De Vloo P, Lee DJ, Dallapiazza RF, Rohani M, Fasano A, Munhoz RP, et al. Deep brain stimulation for pantothenate kinase-associated neurodegeneration: a meta-analysis. Mov Disord. 2019;34:264-73.
80. Brüggemann N, Kühn A, Schneider SA, Kamm C, Wolters A, Krause P, et al. Short- and long-term outcome of chronic pallidal neurostimulation in monogenic isolated dystonia. Neurology. 2015;84:895-90.
81. Rodrigues FB, Duarte GS, Prescott D, Ferreira J, Costa J. Deep brain stimulation for dystonia. Cochrane Database Syst Rev. 2019;1(1):CD012405.

CHAPTER 5

Expanding Indications of Botulinum Neurotoxin in Movement Disorders

Jacky Ganguly, Supriyo Choudhury, Hrishikesh Kumar

ABSTRACT

Botulinum toxin (BoNT), also known as botulinum neurotoxin, despite being the one of most potent biologic toxins, is one of the safest treatment options in clinical practice. In the field of movement disorders, the therapeutic spectrum of BoNT has vastly expanded in the last few decades, incorporating several newer indications including different tremor syndromes, parkinsonism, dyskinesia, focal spasms, myoclonus, and tics. Precise muscle targeting using electromyography (EMG) or ultrasonography (USG) and individualized dosing strategy with kinematic guidance have indicated a potential expansion of the therapeutic indications of BoNT in the coming years.

Keywords: Botulinum toxin, Movement disorders.

INTRODUCTION

Botulinum toxin (BoNT), also known as botulinum neurotoxin, acts at the presynaptic cholinergic nerve terminal by cleaving and inactivating SNARE proteins (SNAP-25 and Syntaxin) responsible for the fusion of acetylcholine vesicles with the presynaptic membrane, inhibiting the release of acetylcholine and preventing the muscle contraction. The paralytic effect of BoNT was initially suggested in 1817 by Justinus Kerner, a German physician, who indicated its potential use in treating hyperkinetic movement disorders and autonomic dysfunction.[1] In the field of movement disorders, BoNT is now widely used in cervical dystonia, blepharospasm, hemifacial spasm, writer's cramp, oromandibular dystonia, spasmodic dysphonia and spasticity. However, in the last few years, the use of BoNT has expanded to different tremor syndromes, motor and non-motor symptoms of Parkinson's disease (PD), atypical parkinsonism, restless leg syndrome, orthostatic tremor, different focal spasms, dyskinesia and tics. The chapter provides an update on the novel applications of BoNT in the treatment of movement disorders.

NEWER INDICATIONS OF BOTULINUM NEUROTOXIN IN MOVEMENT DISORDERS

Essential Tremor

Many patients with essential tremor (ET) fail to respond or develop side effects to conventional treatment like propranolol or primidone. Deep brain stimulation (DBS) surgery targeting ventralis intermediate (VIM) nucleus of thalamus carries its demerits of being invasive and risk of developing ataxia. In this regard, electromyography (EMG)-guided (Yale method) or kinematic/sensor-guided (Western University method) BoNT-A injection to muscles responsible for wrist, shoulder, and elbow movements (total customized dose 30–200 U of EMG-guided BoNT-A injection per patient) can improve tremor amplitude and upper limb function, with or without mild, nontroublesome weakness in the targeted muscles:[2,3]

- *For wrist (5–20 U per muscle, one injection site)*: Extensor carpi radialis (ECR), extensor carpi ulnaris (ECU), flexor carpi radialis (FCR), flexor carpi ulnaris (FCU), pronator quadratus (PQ), pronator teres (PT), and supinator.
- *For shoulder (10–40 U per muscle, 1–3 injection sites)*: Deltoid, latissimus dorsi, pectoralis major, supraspinatus, and teres major
- *For elbow (15–40 U per muscle, two injection sites)*: Biceps brachii, brachialis, and triceps brachii.

During kinematic tremor assessment, patients perform three trials of six scripted tasks:[4]

1. *Rest-1*: Arm in the lap with the palm facing upward.
2. *Rest-2*: Arm supported with palm facing inward.
3. *Posture-1*: Arms outstretched with palms facing downward.
4. *Posture-2*: Arms outstretched with palms facing inward.
5. *Load-1*: Holding an empty cup in front of the chest, elbow flexed.
6. *Load-2*: Holding a cup with a 1-pound weight in front of the chest, elbow flexed.

Kinematic assessment of tremor facilitates individualized injection parameters during BoNT-A therapy to improve functional ability in patients with ET, while targeting the most disabling side or even bilaterally.[5] Previous studies using a standard nonpersonalized protocol (without kinematic guidance) targeting FCR, FCU (15–30 U each) and ECR, and ECU (10–20 U each) also showed improvement in tremor amplitude, but with more wrist and hand weakness.[6]

For clinical assessment, upper limb tremor can be examined in four common plains of movement to ease muscle selection for EMG-guided toxin injection.

1. *Forearm pronation-supination (10 U onabotulinumtoxinA each)*: PT, supinator, and PQ.
2. *Wrist flexion-extension (10–15 U onabotulinumtoxinA each)*: ECR, ECU, FCR, and FCU.
3. *Shoulder internal-external rotation (wing-beating) (10–30 U onabotulinumtoxinA each)*: Teres major and infraspinatus.
4. *Elbow flexion-extension (10–15 U onabotulinumtoxinA each)*: Triceps, brachioradialis, and biceps.

Isolated or Essential Head Tremor

Isolated head tremor as a part of essential tremor syndrome is often refractory to oral therapy. Recently, Marques et al. have demonstrated the beneficial effect of EMG-guided botulinum toxin injection to bilateral splenius capitis (75 IU on each side on day 0 and repeated either in the same dose or increased to 100 IU on week 12) in a large multicentric placebo-controlled trial in such patients.[7]

Parkinson's Disease Tremor

Tremor treatment in PD is often challenging with dopaminergic medication and may require a much higher dose. Anticholinergics cannot be used in all these patients because of their side effects. Kinematic-guided BoNT-A therapy can be beneficial for such patients.[3] Tremor in PD patients should be evaluated in the ON state to assess the refractoriness to ongoing therapies. Kinematic analysis needs to be performed in multiple degrees of freedom (DOF) for each joint—

(1) flexion-extension (F/E), radial-ulnar (R/U) deviations, and pronation-supination (P/S) for the wrist, (2) F/E for the elbow, and (3) F/E, abduction-adduction (A/A) deviations for the shoulder.[8] FCR, FCU, ECR, ECU, PT, PQ, supinator, pectoralis major, deltoid, teres major, supraspinatus, biceps, and triceps are the muscles being targeted. Compared to ET tremor, PD tremor is predominantly distal and thus wrist flexors are commonly more targeted during toxin injection, while muscles around the elbow like the biceps and triceps are mostly spared. On average, each upper limb requires 68–100 units of onabotulinumtoxinA which has been shown to improve the tremor subscore of the UPDRS scale.[9]

Jaw Tremor in Parkinson's Disease

Jaw tremor in PD is commonly vertical up-and-down movement and often refractory to conventional treatment. 30–100 unit of BoNT-A in each masseter muscle (divided between two sites) is helpful in improving the tremor.[10]

Other Motor Symptoms of Parkinson's Disease

Foot and Toe Dystonia

Foot and toe dystonia is seen in PD during OFF state (especially during early morning OFF, often painful) or it can be exercise-induced, more common in early onset genetic PD. EMG-guided BoNT-A therapy can be effective in such cases.

Common patterns and muscles to target are:[11]

- *Great toe extension or striatal toe*: Extensor hallucis longus (EHL).
- *Flexion of other toes or toe-curling*: Flexor digitorum longus and brevis (FDL and FDB)
- *Inversion and/or supination of the foot*: Tibialis posterior (TP), gastrocnemius, and soleus.

Postural Abnormalities in Parkinson's Disease

Excessive truncal anteflexion (camptocormia), often associated with lateral bending (Pisa syndrome), is common in PD. CT/USG and EMG-guided BoNT-A injection to rectus abdominis and iliopsoas (500–800 U in a session) has shown good outcomes for camptocormia, though the response is variable.[12] Bilateral external oblique injection (75–90 U on each side) has also shown a beneficial response under ultrasonic guidance.[13]

An ipsilateral paraspinal injection is needed for Pisa syndrome. EMG/ultrasound-guided 100–300 U BoNT-A is used based on clinical assessment on standing posture and hyperactivity noted in EMG.[14] If EMG hyperactivity is noted bilaterally, the most active side is injected. MRI evaluation can be done to rule out muscle atrophy ipsilateral to the bending side, which can potentially worsen the lateral bending.

Freezing of Gait

Botulinum toxin type-A injection in the medial and lateral head of gastrocnemius and soleus (unilateral/bilateral) of total 100–300 unit/leg has been tried in few studies to improve freezing of gait (FOG) in PD; however, the results are conflicting.[15,16] Another study showed some positive response with injecting tensor fasciae latae bilaterally (50 unit/leg).[17]

Non-motor Symptoms of Parkinson's Disease

Sialorrhea

Sialorrhea or excessive drooling is often a bothersome symptom in patients with PD. It occurs mainly because of swallowing dysfunction due to lingual bradykinesia, oropharyngeal dysphagia, upper esophageal dysmotility and flexed head posture, all leading to impaired salivary clearance.[18] BoNT-A injection (with or without USG guidance) of around 30–40 U in each parotid gland (20–30 U in the upper lobe above the angle of mandible and 10 U in the lower lobe below the angle of mandible) and 10–20 U in each submandibular gland (medial to the midpoint of a line joining the mandibular angle to the tip of the chin along the mandible) is beneficial in controlling sialorrhea.[18,19]

Overactive Bladder

Detrusor hyperactivity or overactive bladder is a common autonomic symptom in PD and multiple system atrophy (MSA), where antimuscarinic or anticholinergic drugs may not be sufficient and can lead to side effects. In refractory cases, cystoscopic injection of BoNT-A into the detrusor muscle (around 100–200 U in multiple sites), ideally done by urologists, can effectively control the symptom.[20,21]

Focal Hyperhidrosis

Sweating dysfunction is frequent in PD, as sudden attacks of profuse sweating. However, few patients may develop focal hyperhidrosis where BoNT-A can be tried.[22]

Focal Dystonia in Atypical Parkinsonism

Progressive Supranuclear Palsy

Botulinum toxin type-A can be tried to treat blepharospasm (pretarsal part of orbicularis oculi) and disabling retrocollis with impairment of swallowing function (bilateral splenius capitis), seen in progressive supranuclear palsy (PSP).[23]

Corticobasal Syndrome

Focal dystonia of hand and fingers along with cortical myoclonus is common in corticobasal syndrome (CBS), where EMG-guided BoNT-A (targeting biceps brachii, brachioradialis, FCR, FCU, ECR, ECU, FDS, and FDP on an individual basis) can temporarily improve upper limb function in the early stage of the disease, whereas in the advanced stage, it can help to reduce pain, maintain hygiene, and prevent contracture.[23]

Multiple System Atrophy

Lower facial dystonia with retraction of the lower lip, especially postlevodopa is common in multiple system atrophy (MSA). BoNT-A targeting orbicularis oris vermilion part has been tried in such patients to reduce lower lip biting and facilitate food intake.[23]

Dystonic Tremor in Spinocerebellar Ataxia Type 12

Postural and action tremor in the upper limbs is common in spinocerebellar ataxia type 12 (SCA12), often associated with dystonic component. BoNT-A has been tried in such dystonic tremor involving neck and arm along with spasmodic dysphonia, that can also be present in SCA12.[24]

Restless Leg Syndrome

Few studies have explored the role of BoNT in restless leg syndrome (RLS). BoNT injection into the muscles reduces the hypersensitivity of motor and sensory systems. BoNT can reduce the discharge of muscle spindles and can reach up to the spinal cord via retrograde transmission and directly influence the spinal cord neurons. Injecting bilateral tibialis anterior (40 U × 2), gastrocnemius (40 U × 2), and biceps femoris (20 U × 2) under EMG guidance has shown a beneficial response.[25] Using lower doses was not found to be effective. Intradermal grid-like injection in each symptomatic zone (250 U per zone) was noted to be ineffective as well.[26] Individualized treatment with 100–300 U in the quadriceps or hamstring and 50–100 U in the gastrocnemius or tibialis posterior has shown better outcomes.[1]

Palatal Myoclonus

Palatal myoclonus (PM) results in elevation and posterior retraction of the soft palate. Essential PM has no definable etiology, whereas symptomatic PM occurs due to pathology in the Guillain-Mollaret triangle. Ear clicks are often present in essential PM and be troublesome. BoNT-A injection to tensor veli palatini under EMG guidance approximately 3–5 mm posterior to the posterior edge of the bony palate (2.5–7.5 U into the lateral soft palate just medial to the pterygoid hamulus and 2.5–3 U into the medial soft palate just lateral to musculus uvulae) can improve the symptoms.[27] If the injection is placed too posteriorly, the posterior fasciculus of the palatopharyngeus can be affected and lead to dysphagia, whereas injecting too anteriorly will involve the anterior fasciculus of the palatopharyngeus.[28] If ear clicks are a predominant symptom, better to inject more dose laterally targeting tensor veli palatini, while more dose to inject medially targeting levator veli palatini if ear clicks are not that prominent.

Spinal Myoclonus

Botulinum toxin type-A has been used in a few patients with focal or segmental spinal myoclonus, involving the neck (splenius capitis, geniohyoid, infrahyoid, and horizontal trapezius) or limbs (quadriceps).[29,30] The toxin can also help in reducing the jerks of propriospinal myoclonus, commonly a functional movement disorder.[31]

Orthostatic Tremor

Orthostatic tremor is classically characterized by tremor in legs while standing, that improves on walking. BoNT-A injection has shown variable response in such cases. Muscles targeted are medial and lateral head of gastrocnemius and tibialis anterior (around 100 units on each side).[32] Future studies with individualized dosing targeting proximal (quadriceps and hamstrings) and distal (tibialis anterior and gastrocnemius-soleus) muscles based on EMG activity can be helpful in this regard.

There is also evidence of a beneficial response with BoNT-A (bilateral masseter 30 × 2) for high-frequency orthostatic jaw tremor.[33]

Palmaris Brevis Spasm

Palmaris brevis spasm syndrome is manifested by spontaneous, recurrent contraction of the palmaris brevis muscle, leading to irregular dimpling over the hypothenar eminence. It has been mostly reported with overuse of computer keyboard, mouse, pipette, vibratory tools, and can even be spontaneous as well. Significant improvement noted with BoNT-A injection in palmaris brevis muscle under EMG guidance (20 units on each side).[34]

Geniospasm

Geniospasm or "trembling chin" is characterized by paroxysmal rhythmic or irregular twitching of the chin and lower lip due to repetitive contractions of the mentalis muscle. It can be hereditary and sometimes even can lead to repeated nocturnal painful tongue bite and lacerations. BoNT-A injection in mentalis muscle (5–30 units on each side) has shown complete resolution of symptoms.[35]

Painful Leg Moving Toes

Painful leg moving toe (PLMT) is often a therapeutic challenge. EMG-guided BoNT-A injection has shown good outcome in some studies. Muscles targeted are abductor digiti minimi (10 units), flexor digiti minimi (10 units), flexor hallucis brevis (25 units), adductor hallucis (25 units), and flexor digitorum brevis (50 units) based on EMG activity.[36,37]

Tardive Orolingual Dyskinesia

Tardive orofacial-lingual-masticatory dyskinesia is common after exposure to neuroleptics and dopamine-receptor blockers like levosulpiride. BoNT has proven to be efficacious in these patients targeting tongue (genioglossus), perioral muscles (incisural or vermilion part of orbicularis oris, risorius, zygomaticus, levator/depressor angularis oris, levator labii superioris alaeque nasi, and levator labii superioris) and sometimes jaw muscles (masseter and medial pterygoid for jaw closing, lateral pterygoid, and digastric for jaw opening) on an individual basis.[38]

Dancing Scapula

Focal dystonic contractions of levator scapulae with rhomboids major and minor lead to rhythmic upward scapular movement with a clicking sound. EMG-guided BoNT injection to levator scapulae (30 units) has shown beneficial outcome for such patients.[39]

Dancing Dorsal Quadrilaterals

Dorsal afferent nerve injury, commonly after upper spine instrumentation, can be associated with repetitive, writhing, and jerky movements with distinctive rotatory component affecting dorsal quadrilateral muscles (trapezius and rhomboids) in upright posture, along with neuropathic pain. EMG-guided BoNT injection to bilateral trapezius and rhomboids (around 300 units) can be helpful in these cases.[40]

Moving Ear Syndrome

Moving ear syndrome (MES) or ear dyskinesia happens due to an involuntary, rhythmic, or semirhythmic contraction of mostly auricularis posterior and sometimes auricularis superior and temporalis muscles. EMG-guided BoNT-A injection in these muscles (dose varies between 10 and 60 units) have shown significant improvement in the movement.[41]

Belly Dancer's Dyskinesia

Belly dancer's dyskinesia is characterized by involuntary writhing movements of the anterior abdominal wall, causing repetitive semirhythmic multidirectional displacements of the umbilicus. USG-/EMG-guided BoNT-A injection to bilateral rectus abdominis muscle (two to three sites on each side, 40–50 unit per site) has been tried in such patients with a good outcome.[42]

Tics

Botulinum toxin type-A has been beneficial in controlling simple motor and vocal tics. Blink (orbicularis oculi pretarsal part), neck turn/extension (sternocleidomastoid and splenius capitis), brow lift (frontalis), sniffing (transverse nasalis), and shoulder shrug (levator scapulae and horizontal trapezius) are the common motor tics where BoNT-A not only reduced the frequency of the tics but also controlled the urge to perform them.[43] BoNT-A injection into vocal cords (2.5 U on each side) under EMG guidance helped to control phonic tics of Tourette syndrome.[44]

CONCLUSION

Botulinum neurotoxin is a safe therapeutic strategy for a variety of hyperkinetic movement disorders. Over the last few decades, the indications are gradually expanding. Recent use of BoNT in tremor syndromes and in various motor and non-motor symptoms of typical or atypical parkinsonism is encouraging. BoNT has been beneficial in managing several focal spasms and dyskinesias, those are otherwise refractory to oral medication. Advanced methods of administration with precise muscle targeting by using EMG and USG, individualized dosing strategy with kinematic guidance and research with novel formulations will further expand the therapeutic spectrum of BoNT in the coming years.

REFERENCES

1. Anandan C, Jankovic J. Botulinum Toxin in Movement Disorders: An Update. Toxins (Basel). 2021;13(1):42.
2. Jog M, Lee J, Scheschonka A, Chen R, Ismail F, Boulias C, et al. Tolerability and Efficacy of Customized IncobotulinumtoxinA Injections for Essential Tremor: A Randomized, Double-Blind, Placebo-Controlled Study. Toxins (Basel). 2020;12(12):807.
3. Mittal SO, Jog M, Lee J, Jabbari B. Novel Botulinum Toxin Injection Protocols for Parkinson Tremor and Essential Tremor—the Yale Technique and Sensor-Based Kinematics Procedure for Safe and Effective Treatment. Tremor Other Hyperkinet Mov (N Y). 2020;10:61.
4. Samotus O, Lee J, Jog M. Developing a Consistent, Reproducible Botulinum Toxin Type A Dosing Method for Upper Limb Tremor by Kinematic Analysis. Toxins (Basel). 2021;13(4):264.
5. Samotus O, Rahimi F, Lee J, Jog M. Functional Ability Improved in Essential Tremor by IncobotulinumtoxinA Injections Using Kinematically Determined Biomechanical Patterns – A New Future. PLoS One. 2016;11(4):e0153739.
6. Brin MF, Lyons KE, Doucette J, Adler CH, Caviness JN, Comella CL, et al. A randomized, double masked, controlled trial of botulinum toxin type A in essential hand tremor. Neurology. 2001;56(11):1523-8.
7. Marques A, Pereira B, Simonetta-Moreau M, Castelnovo G, De Verdal M, Fluchère F, et al. Trial of Botulinum Toxin for Isolated or Essential Head Tremor. N Engl J Med. 2023;389(19):1753-65.
8. Samotus O, Mahdi Y, Jog M. Real-World Longitudinal Experience of Botulinum Toxin Therapy for Parkinson and Essential Tremor. Toxins (Basel). 2022;14(8):557.
9. Eslamian F, Dolatkhah N, Fallah L, Jahanjoo F, Toopchizadeh V, Talebi M. Effectiveness of Botulinum Toxin on Hand Tremor Intensity and Upper Limb Function in Patients with Parkinson's Disease: Results of a Systematic Review. Tremor Other Hyperkinet Mov (N Y). 2023;13:27.
10. Schneider SA, Edwards MJ, Cordivari C, Macleod WN, Bhatia KP. Botulinum toxin a may be efficacious as treatment for jaw tremor in Parkinson's disease. Mov Disord. 2006;21(10):1722-4.
11. Rieu I, Degos B, Castelnovo G, Vial C, Durand E, Pereira B, et al. Incobotulinum toxin A in Parkinson's disease with foot dystonia: A double-blind randomized trial. Parkinsonism Relat Disord. 2018;46:9-15.
12. Srivanitchapoom P, Hallett M. Camptocormia in Parkinson's disease: definition, epidemiology, pathogenesis and treatment modalities. J Neurol Neurosurg Psychiatry. 2016;87(1):75-85.
13. Todo H, Yamasaki H, Ogawa G, Nishida K, Futamura N, Funakawa I. Injection of Onabotulinum Toxin A into the Bilateral External Oblique Muscle Attenuated Camptocormia: A Prospective Open-Label Study in Six Patients with Parkinson's Disease. Neurol Ther. 2018;7(2):365-71.
14. Etoom M, Alwardat M, Aburub AS, Lena F, Fabbrizo R, Modugno N, et al. Therapeutic interventions for Pisa syndrome in idiopathic Parkinson's disease. A Scoping Systematic Review. Clin Neurol Neurosurg. 2020;198:106242.
15. Giladi N, Gurevich T, Shabtai H, Paleacu D, Simon ES. The effect of botulinum toxin injections to the calf muscles on freezing of gait in parkinsonism: a pilot study. J Neurol. 2001;248(7):572-6.
16. Gurevich T, Peretz C, Moore O, Weizmann N, Giladi N. The effect of injecting botulinum toxin type a into the calf muscles on freezing of gait in Parkinson's disease: A double blind placebo-controlled pilot study. Mov Disord. 2007;22(6):880-3.
17. Vastik M, Hok P, Hlustik P, Otruba P, Tüdös Z, Kanovsky P. Botulinum toxin treatment of freezing of gait in Parkinson's disease patients as reflected in functional magnetic resonance imaging of leg movement. Neuro Endocrinol Lett. 2016;37(2):147-53.
18. Mehta S, Lal V. Treatment of sialorrhea in Parkinson's disease. Ann Mov Disord. 2022;5(3):153.
19. Ruiz-Roca JA, Pons-Fuster E, Lopez-Jornet P. Effectiveness of the Botulinum Toxin for Treating Sialorrhea in Patients with Parkinson's Disease: A Systematic Review. J Clin Med. 2019;8(3):317.
20. Hajebrahimi S, Chapple CR, Pashazadeh F, Salehi-Pourmehr H. Management of neurogenic bladder in patients with Parkinson's disease: A systematic review. Neurourol Urodyn. 2019;38(1):31-62.
21. Giannantoni A, Rossi A, Mearini E, Del Zingaro M, Porena M, Berardelli A. Botulinum Toxin A for Overactive Bladder and Detrusor Muscle Overactivity in Patients With Parkinson's Disease and Multiple System Atrophy. J Urol. 2009;182(4):1453-7.
22. Jost WH. Use of Botulinum Neurotoxin in Parkinson's Disease: A Critical Appraisal. Toxins (Basel). 2021;13(2):87.
23. Müller J, Wenning GK, Wissel J, Seppi K, Poewe W. Botulinum toxin treatment in atypical parkinsonian disorders associated with disabling focal dystonia. J Neurol. 2002;249(3):300-4.

24. Ganos C, Saifee TA, Kassavetis P, Erro R, Batla A, Cordivari C, et al. Dystonic Tremor and Spasmodic Dysphonia in Spinocerebellar Ataxia Type 12. Mov Disord Clin Pract. 2014;1(1):79-81.
25. Mittal S, Machado D, Richardson D, Dubey D, Jabbari B. Botulinum Toxin in Restless Legs Syndrome—A Randomized Double-Blind Placebo-Controlled Crossover Study. Toxins (Basel). 2018;10(10):401.
26. Ghorayeb I, Bénard A, Vivot A, Tison F, Burbaud P. A phase II, open-label, non-comparative study of Botulinum toxin in Restless Legs Syndrome. Sleep Med. 2012;13(10):1313-6.
27. Anis MM, Pollak N. Treatment of Palatal Myoclonus with Botulinum Toxin Injection. Case Rep Otolaryngol. 2013;2013:1-3.
28. Chitkara A, Cultrara A, Blitzer A. Palatal myoclonus: treatment with botulinum toxin. Oper Tech Otolayngol Head Neck Surg. 2004;15(2):114-7.
29. Lagueny A, Tison F, Burbaud P, Masson G Le, Kien P. Stimulus-sensitive spinal segmental myoclonus improved with injections of botulinum toxin type A. Mov Disord. 1999;14(1):182-5.
30. Polo KB, Jabbari B. Effectiveness of botulinum toxin type A against painful limb myoclonus of spinal cord origin. Mov Disord. 1994;9(2):233-5.
31. van der Salm SMA, Erro R, Cordivari C, Edwards MJ, Koelman JH, van den Ende T, et al. Propriospinal myoclonus: clinical reappraisal and review of literature. Neurology. 2014;83(20):1862-70.
32. Kim SH, Han JY, Song MK, Choi IS, Park HK. Orthostatic tremor after knee contusion without head trauma: A rare case report. Turk J Phys Med Rehabil. 2023;1(1):111-5.
33. Gonzalez-Alegre P, Kelkar P, Rodnitzky RL. Isolated high-frequency jaw tremor relieved by botulinum toxin injections. Mov Disord. 2006;21(7):1049-50.
34. Ganguly J, Pandita N, Banerjee S, Mukherjee S, Singh N, Basu P, et al. Palmaris brevis spasm syndrome: The treatable hypothenar dimpling. Ann Mov Disord. 2024.
35. Hull M, Parnes M. Effective Treatment of Geniospasm: Case Series and Review of the Literature. Tremor Other Hyperkin Mov (N Y). 2020;10:31.
36. Rodriguez RL, Fernandez HH. Sustained benefit of painful legs moving toes syndrome with botulinum toxin type A. J Clin Neurosci. 2013;20(7):1031-2.
37. Schoffer K. Painful leg moving toes treated with botulinum toxin type A: A video report. Mov Disord. 2010;25(6):784-5.
38. Rapaport A, Sadeh M, Stein D, Levine J, Sirota P, Mosheva T, et al. Botulinum toxin for the treatment of oro-facial-lingual-masticatory tardive dyskinesia. Mov Disord. 2000;15(2):352-5.
39. Elavarasi A, Goyal V, Samal P. Dancing scapula: The missed movement. Ann Indian Acad Neurol. 2019;22(2):218.
40. Lizarraga KJ, Thompson PD, Moore HP, Mizraji G, Gershanik OS, Singer C, et al. Dancing Dorsal Quadrilaterals: A Novel Peripherally Induced Movement Disorder. JAMA Neurol. 2019;76(3):351-4.
41. Yahya V, Chavez RC, Campiglio L, Zardoni M, Priori A. Moving Ear Syndrome: A rare and treatable phenomenon. Parkinsonism Relat Disord. 2024;122:106921.
42. Alshubaili A, Abou-Al-Shaar H, Santhamoorthy P, Attia H, Bohlega S. Ultrasound-guided botulinum toxin A injection in the treatment of belly dancer's dyskinesia. BMC Neurol. 2016;16(1):226.
43. Rath JJG, Tavy DLJ, Wertenbroek AAACM, van Woerkom TCAM, de Bruijn SFTM. Botulinum toxin type A in simple motor tics: Short-term and long-term treatment-effects. Parkinsonism Relat Disord. 2010;16(7):478-81.
44. Porta M, Maggioni G, Ottaviani F, Schindler A. Treatment of phonic tics in patients with Tourette's syndrome using botulinum toxin type A. Neurol Sci. 2004;24(6):420-3.

CHAPTER

6

Drug-induced Movement Disorders

P Vijayashankar, G Balaji, U Meenakshisundaram

ABSTRACT

The movement disorders caused by therapeutic or illicit drugs could phenomenologically be hypo or hyperkinetic, presenting acute or late after exposure to the offending drugs (even during withdrawal of neuroleptics), and could range from a subtle finding to a life-threatening event. This chapter is a brief description of the approach to common drug-induced movement disorders emphasizing more on the management of tardive syndromes. The challenges in management compel a preventive approach ensuring the use of the offending agents strictly limited to appropriate indication, doses, and duration.

Keywords: Offending drugs, Drug induced movement disorders, Challenges, Neuroleptics, Management.

INTRODUCTION

Drug-induced movement disorders (DIMD) are significant and treatable conditions that can manifest as acute, subacute, or chronic, with severity ranging from mild-to-severe, and in some cases, potentially life-threatening. The severity of symptoms does not necessarily correlate with the duration of drug exposure. Common drugs implicated in these disorders include antidepressants, antipsychotics, prokinetics, antiemetics, antiepileptics, antimicrobials, antiarrhythmics, and mood stabilizers, among others. These disorders encompass a range of movement abnormalities, including dyskinesias, dystonia, parkinsonism, tremor, chorea, akathisia, tics, and ataxia, or a combination thereof. While the presentation is often straightforward, in some cases a thorough review of past medical records and over-the-counter medications may be necessary to identify the etiology. It is crucial to consider DIMD in any recent-onset movement disorder to enable timely intervention.

ACUTE AND TARDIVE PRESENTATIONS

Acute DIMD can appear within minutes to days after drug administration and may present as either focal or generalized disturbances. A common manifestation is tardive dyskinesia (TD), characterized by involuntary twitching or writhing movements, typically involving the perioral region, tongue, and face. This condition can result in repetitive chewing or eating movements resembling those of a rabbit (known as rabbit syndrome) and may impair speech, with less frequent involvement of the limbs and trunk.

Additionally, TD can be associated with the development of other movement disorders, including akathisia, tremor, neuroleptic malignant syndrome, serotonin syndrome, parkinsonism-hyperpyrexia disorder, and acute dystonic reactions. Neuroleptic malignant syndrome, malignant catatonia, serotonin syndrome, acute chorea-ballism, and status dystonicus some of which are life-threatening presentations. Tardive DIMD occur either during exposure or within weeks of stopping a drug and are present for at least one month.[1,2] The minimum duration of exposure to the drug before developing movements is 3 months, or 1 month in adults aged over 60 years.

Table 1 is a summary of movement disorders caused by therapeutic drugs.[3]

TABLE 1: Summary of movement disorders caused by therapeutic drugs.[3]

Movement disorder	Implicated drugs
Akathisia	• Dopamine receptor-blocking drugs • Selective serotonin reuptake inhibitors • Antiepileptics
Tremor	• Selective serotonin reuptake inhibitors • Lithium • Tricyclic antidepressants • Antiepileptics (e.g., valproate) • Bronchodilators • Amiodarone • Immunosuppressive drugs (tacrolimus and ciclosporin)
Serotonin syndrome (usually due to overdose or combinations of serotoninergic drugs)	• Selective serotonin reuptake inhibitors • Serotonin noradrenaline reuptake inhibitors • Tricyclic antidepressants • Monoamine oxidase inhibitors • Lithium • Linezolid • Opioids (pethidine, tramadol, propentadol) • Antiepileptics (valproate, and lamotrigine) • St John's wort
Acute dystonic reaction	• Dopamine receptor-blocking drugs (e.g., antipsychotics and metoclopramide) • Selective serotonin reuptake inhibitors • Opioids • Methylphenidate • Rivastigmine • Albendazole • Gabapentin • Cetirizine • Foscarnet • Quinine • Propofol • Sevoflurane

Continued

Continued

Movement disorder	Implicated drugs
Neuroleptic malignant syndrome	• Antipsychotics (e.g., haloperidol, fluphenazine, and chlorpromazine) • Prochlorperazine • Metoclopramide • Droperidol • Promethazine • Tetrabenazine • Lithium
Parkinsonism	• Dopamine receptor-blocking drugs (e.g., antipsychotics) • Calcium channel antagonists (e.g., flunarizine and cinnarizine) • Antiepileptics (e.g., phenytoin, valproate, and levetiracetam) • Antidepressants (e.g., selective serotonin reuptake inhibitors, and monoamine oxidase inhibitors) • Lithium • Chemotherapeutic drugs (e.g., cytosine arabinoside, cyclophosphamide, vincristine, adriamycin, doxorubicin, paclitaxel, and etoposide) • Immunosuppressive drugs (e.g., ciclosporin, and tacrolimus) • Toxins [e.g., 1-methyl-4-phenyl-1,2,3,6-tetrahydropyridine (MPTP), organophosphate pesticides, manganese, methanol, cyanide, carbon monoxide, and carbon disulfide]
Tardive drug-induced movement disorders	• Antipsychotics • Antiemetics (e.g., metoclopramide)

Table 2 is a summary of movement disorders caused by illicit drugs.

Is it drug-induced Parkinsonism (DIP)?

A familiar question that arises when patients on neuroleptics or such offending drugs present with parkinsonian features is whether it is DIP or unmasking of an underlying idiopathic Parkinson's disease (PD). The presence of nonmotor symptoms such as anosmia/rapid eye movement (REM) behavioral disorders and response to stopping the offending drug could offer more clues than the motor symptoms (except gait freezing) as the motor features of DIP and PD can be identical. Symptoms in the majority of patients emerge within 3 months of initiation of neuroleptics although it can manifest within days of medication initiation. A second peak of symptom onset at 12 months of exposure has been reported, mainly with the use of calcium channel blockers **(Table 2)**.

Although DIP symptoms may persist up to 18 months, a majority (two-thirds) of patients recover within 7 weeks. Alternatively, when symptoms persist and worsen with time, idiopathic PD which was preclinical at the time of neuroleptic exposure should be suspected. Dopamine active transporter (DAT) scans evaluate presynaptic terminal density whereas dopamine-receptor blocking agents exert their action via postsynaptic receptors and DIP patients have negative DAT scans.

TABLE 2: Summary of movement disorders caused by illicit drugs.

Drug	Movement disorder
Cocaine	• Choreoathetosis (chorea and dystonia, also known as "crack dancing") • Stereotypies • Tremor • Myoclonust
Amphetamines	• Punding (purposeless and repetitive behaviors) • Tremor • Dystonia • Choreoathetosis • Orolingual dyskinesia
3,4-methylenedioxymethamphetamine (MDMA)	• Serotonin syndrome • Parkinsonism
Opioids	• Myoclonus

NEUROLEPTIC MALIGNANT SYNDROME

Neuroleptic malignant syndrome (NMS) is an idiosyncratic complication caused by antipsychotic drugs in virtually all cases within 30 days of initiation or with the withdrawal of dopaminergic agents.[4] Clinical presentation of NMS is not identical always and usually starts with the unexplainable collection of symptoms like tremors, muscle cramps, unstable blood pressure (BP), and disturbance of mental status—anxiety, agitation, delirium, and coma. Sometimes, hyperpyrexia can be delayed for more than 24 hours, which can lead to diagnostic confusion. Laboratories [creatine phosphokinase (CPK) levels are usually above 1,000 IU/L] help in the exclusion of other serious conditions mimicking NMS such as Parkinsonism-hyperpyrexia disorder.

SEROTONIN SYNDROME

For serotonin syndrome, a diagnosis of exclusion needs to be considered in patients on drugs mentioned in **Table 1** presenting with delirium, anxiety, dilated pupil, autonomic dysfunction, vomiting, diarrhea, hyperreflexia, myoclonus, ocular clonus, tremor, akathisia, and with positive Babinski sign.

ACUTE DYSTONIA

Acute sustained dystonic spasm of craniocervical muscles is typical, but oculogyric crises, truncal spasm causing opisthotonos, or limb dystonia can also occur. They are more common among younger patients and seen with prokinetics (prides) and other dopamine receptor-blocking drugs. Acute laryngeal dystonia can be life-threatening due to airway obstruction and requires emergency medical care. Treatment consists of stopping the offending drug along with a short course of anticholinergics and benzodiazepines treatment.

WHEN TO SUSPECT DRUG-INDUCED MOVEMENT DISORDERS

To suspect DIMD in a clinical setting, consider the following indicators: The onset of symptoms immediately after starting a new medication or increasing the dose of an existing one. Look for associated movement disorders such as akathisia, orofacial dyskinesia, or tardive syndromes (TS), including symmetrical Parkinsonism with tremors, sudden truncal dystonia, oculogyric crisis, and acute dystonia. For patients already prescribed dopamine receptor antagonists, it is important to review their medication history carefully when DIMD is suspected. For patients currently taking dopamine receptor antagonists, it is advisable to review their medication history thoroughly when DIMD is suspected.

MANAGEMENT OF DRUG-INDUCED MOVEMENT DISORDERS

Managing DIMD is particularly challenging and is often inappropriately managed. The most common drugs are dopamine receptor-blocking agents (DRBA), specifically antipsychotics and antiemetics. A meta-analysis of 41 studies since 2000 investigated the prevalence of TD in patients treated with first-generation antipsychotics (FGAs) and second-generation antipsychotics (SGAs). The analysis revealed a significantly lower mean TD prevalence in patients receiving SGAs (21%) than those on FGAs (30%). The initial approach involves carefully discontinuing or reducing the dose of the offending DRBA without exacerbating the underlying psychotic symptoms. Gradual tapering is recommended, as abrupt withdrawal can worsen TD. Although TD may improve several weeks or months after discontinuation, more than 50% of cases remain irreversible. The remission rate of TS varies between 2 and 12% after up to 4 years of DRBA discontinuation or dose reduction. The risk factors for TS include older age, female gender, schizoaffective disorders, prolonged antipsychotic use, high antipsychotic doses, dementia, diabetes mellitus, human immunodeficiency virus (HIV) infection, intellectual disability, brain damage, and use of anticholinergics. Racial disparities, such as higher dosages prescribed to African Americans compared to other Americans, may also contribute to risk.

For patients with ongoing psychotic symptoms who develop TD while on FGAs, it is essential to reassess the severity of symptoms. When indicated, a safer and more effective alternative medication should be considered. Prescribing the lowest effective dose of an SGA with a low risk of TD for a short duration can help manage symptoms. However, while withdrawing all antipsychotics reduces the severity of Parkinsonism, switching from FGAs to SGAs does not necessarily improve TD.

Clozapine, quetiapine, and iloperidone, known for their weak affinity for dopamine receptors, carry a lower risk of triggering or exacerbating TD. Clozapine is particularly favored for its minimal impact on dopamine receptors, although it requires regular blood count monitoring due to potential rare bone marrow toxicity. Quetiapine and olanzapine, lacking this risk, are more commonly prescribed for managing TD and seldom induce extrapyramidal disorders. This strategy resembles near-complete cessation of medication, often referred to as "passive healing", with the hope of reversing TS upon discontinuation of dopamine receptor-blocking drugs. However, many patients cannot discontinue these medications due to treatment failure. In such cases, switching to aripiprazole is often advised, though its effectiveness in this scenario remains uncertain.

New evidence along with existing guideline recommendations suggest deutetrabenazine and valbenazine are established as effective treatments for TD (Level A) and are recommended for use. Clonazepam and *Ginkgo biloba* likely improve TD (Level B) and should be considered as treatment options. Amantadine and tetrabenazine may be considered for TD treatment (Level C). Pallidal deep brain stimulation (DBS) potentially improves TD and could be considered for cases of refractory TD (Level C). Insufficient evidence exists to support or refute the treatment of TD by withdrawing causative agents or switching from typical to atypical DRBAs (Level U).[1]

Vesicular Monoamine Transporter Type 2 Inhibitors

Vesicular monoamine transporter type 2 (VMAT2) inhibitors are the primary symptomatic treatment for managing moderate-to-severe TD. These medications can be administered with or without concurrent antipsychotic therapy. Three VMAT2 inhibitors that are Food and Drug Administration (FDA) approved for treating TD are tetrabenazine, valbenazine, and deutetrabenazine.

Tetrabenazine

Tetrabenazine is supported by the most robust evidence among the three drugs. Two Class III studies demonstrated a significant reduction in the abnormal involuntary movement scale (AIMS) scores (>50%) according to both self-ratings and blinded videotape raters. Conversely, a Class IV study found no improvement in AIMS scores following a 6-week trial of tetrabenazine in 10 elderly patients with TD.[5] The medication is typically initiated at a dose of 12.5 mg daily for 1 week, then increased by 12.5 mg increments every 5–7 days to an effective dose range of 75–150 mg daily, divided into three doses due to its short half-life.

Valbenazine

Valbenazine, a prodrug of the active α-dihydrotetrabenazine (DH-TBZ) isomers, is designed for slow metabolism to minimize peak plasma concentrations and reduce variability among individuals. It has a long half-life of approximately 20 hours and is administered once daily. The initial dose is 40 mg, which can be increased to a maximum of 80 mg daily after 1 or more weeks. The KINECT 4 study reported that by week 4, 55% of participants experienced clinically meaningful improvement, which increased to 97% by week 48. A total of 86% of participants achieved ≥50% improvement in AIMS scores, with TD improvement sustained throughout the treatment period. The mean AIMS total score decreased by 10.5 points from baseline to week 48. Additionally, over 88% of participants demonstrated significant improvement in the clinical global impression of change-TD (CGI-TD) and patient global impression of change (PGIC) ratings by week 48.[6] The J-KINECT study also demonstrated significant improvement in CGI-TD scores at week 6 in both the 80 mg (2.8) and 40 mg (3.0) groups compared to placebo.[7]

Deutetrabenazine

Deutetrabenazine, a deuterated form of tetrabenazine, offers the advantage of slower metabolite breakdown, resulting in a longer duration of action. Treatment typically starts at 6 mg twice daily, with weekly increases of 6 mg/day to a maximum dose of 48 mg/day. Deutetrabenazine's pharmacokinetics are less influenced by the 2D6 genotype, eliminating the need for general genotyping recommended for patients taking more than 50 mg/day of tetrabenazine. A Phase 3, double-blind, placebo-controlled study (AIM-TD) evaluating fixed doses of 12 mg,

24 mg, or 36 mg/day in 298 patients with TD showed significant changes in AIMS scores for the 24 mg (-1.8 ± 0.60, $p = 0.003$) and 36 mg (-1.9 ± 0.58, $p = 0.001$) groups compared to placebo.[8] Similarly, the ARM-TD study indicated that deutetrabenazine was well tolerated, with significant reduction in abnormal movements.[9]

Comparative and Side Effects

Direct comparisons between the three VMAT2 inhibitors have not been conducted. Valbenazine and deutetrabenazine do not show superiority over each other. However, valbenazine and deutetrabenazine offer the convenience of once or twice-daily dosing due to their longer half-lives. Valbenazine is administered once daily, whereas deutetrabenazine is given twice daily and offers flexibility with multiple dosing options. As spontaneous remission can occur occasionally, gradual dose reduction should be considered. This sustained pharmacokinetic profile may contribute to their reduced side effects, particularly avoiding depression and Parkinsonism when compared to tetrabenazine. Common side effects shared by all three VMAT2 inhibitors include somnolence and fatigue, which may improve with slow titration. Less common side effects include akathisia, Parkinsonism, depression, and tremors.

Benzodiazepines

Benzodiazepines, such as clonazepam, can be beneficial for managing mild TD by alleviating mild dyskinesias and associated anxiety. However, their long-term efficacy is limited due to the development of tolerance and diminished effectiveness over time. The initial dosage is typically 0.5 mg daily, with incremental increases of 0.5 mg every 5 days based on patient response and tolerance, up to a maximum of 3–4 mg/day. Common side effects include sedation, confusion, and ataxia.

Amantadine

Amantadine may serve as an adjunct therapy when continuation of antipsychotics is necessary. It can be administered up to a dose of 300 mg/day. This medication can help manage symptoms when discontinuing antipsychotics is not an option.

Anticholinergics

Anticholinergics have been used to treat TD based on their effectiveness in managing idiopathic dystonia. However, they generally worsen the classical orofacial syndrome and increase the risk of its development. In the largest TD cohort study, out of 54 patients treated with anticholinergics, mild benefit was observed in 16 patients, moderate benefit in six, and marked benefit in two.[10] Trihexyphenidyl, administered at doses ranging from 6–36 mg daily, has shown amelioration of tardive dystonia in some case reports, particularly when used in conjunction with the discontinuation or reduction of DRBAs.

Baclofen

Several trials have produced mixed results regarding baclofen's efficacy in treating TD. One study reported mild benefits in four patients and moderate benefits in one out of nine patients. Other case reports indicate mild-to-modest improvements with doses ranging from 60 to 80 mg/day. One patient experienced significant improvement in dystonia with an intrathecal baclofen infusion of 100 µg/day after failing to respond to oral medications, botulinum toxin, and neurotomy.[11]

Ginkgo biloba Extract

Ginkgo biloba is used as a presumed antioxidative agent. A Chinese study found that *Ginkgo biloba* extract significantly reduced AIMS scores, with 51% of the treatment group achieving a ≥30% reduction in AIMS scores compared to 5.1% of the placebo group.[12]

Other Treatments

There is insufficient evidence to support or refute the use of acetazolamide, bromocriptine, thiamine, vitamin E, vitamin B6, selegiline, olanzapine, melatonin, nifedipine, fluperlapine, sulpiride, flupenthixol, thiopropazate, haloperidol, levetiracetam, quetiapine, ziprasidone, sertindole, aripiprazole, buspirone, Yi-Gan San, biperiden discontinuation, botulinum toxin type A, electroconvulsive therapy, alpha-methyldopa, and reserpine as treatments for TD. Electroconvulsive therapy has been extensively documented to enhance mobility in patients with Parkinson's disease, yet its impact on choreic disorders, dystonia, and TS remains uncertain.

Botulinum Toxin

Botulinum toxin is frequently used to treat TS, though no double-blind, controlled trials have been conducted. Kiriakakis et al. reported improvements in 83% of patients with tardive cervical dystonia and 86% of those with tardive blepharospasm.[10] An open-label study involving 34 patients with TD who received botulinum toxin injections showed moderate-to-marked improvement in 29 out of 38 treated body regions.[13] In a comparison study of botulinum toxin type A between idiopathic cervical dystonia (ICD) and tardive cervical dystonia, 149 ICD patients and seven TD patients experienced similar severity improvements. However, the TD group required a higher average dose (287 vs. 220 units).[14] Another study with 92 idiopathic and 24 tardive oromandibular dystonia patients confirmed moderate benefits of botulinum toxin. This study found no differences in dose and efficacy between the groups when treating the masseters, geniohyoid, digastric, and mylohyoid muscles.[15]

Deep Brain Stimulation

Deep brain stimulation is beneficial for patients with persistent and troublesome dyskinesia that is refractory to conventional medications (Level C). The globus pallidus internus (GPi) is a well-established DBS target for Parkinson's disease and dystonia, effectively controlling levodopa-induced dyskinesias and refractory TD.

The GPi DBS is considered a safe and promising treatment, showing 30–90% improvement on disease-specific scales over up to 7 years.[16] Some studies have explored subthalamic nucleus (STN) DBS for TD with beneficial effects, but GPi DBS remains more commonly studied and used. DBS is typically considered for patients with severe, disabling symptoms unresponsive to other treatments, requiring careful patient selection and assessment for eligibility.

The French stimulation for tardive dyskinesia (STARDY) study reported 50% motor improvement in 10 patients after 6 months of GPi DBS.[17] Another study showed up to a 70% reduction in involuntary movements and about a 90% reduction in dystonic symptoms after 5–14 years of pallidal DBS.[16] These patients experienced significant suppression of phasic and/or tremulous dystonic movements with good outcomes.

While a few patients with isolated dystonia achieved disease remission, many experienced reappearance and even rebound of TD after discontinuing stimulation. Importantly, DBS did not aggravate underlying psychiatric comorbidities, suggesting GPi DBS may be useful for pharmacologically refractory severe TD in patients with stable psychiatric conditions.

Ablative Surgeries

Evidence for pallidotomy in treating TS is limited. However, bilateral pallidotomy in severe TD showed significant improvements, reducing the motor score from 76 to 21 and the disability score from 22 to 4 on the Burke-Fahn-Marsden Dystonia Rating Scale (BFMDRS).[18] Another case report demonstrated a 95% improvement in motor BFMDRS score following bilateral pallidotomy after DBS hardware rejection.[19] Additionally, staged bilateral pallidotomy resolved tardive camptocormia and life-threatening tardive jaw opening dystonia in separate patients.

MANAGEMENT OF NEUROLEPTIC MALIGNANT SYNDROME AND SEROTONIN SYNDROME

Recognizing and promptly treating NMS and serotonin syndrome is crucial. Treatment consists of immediate withdrawal of the offending agent and supportive medical therapy. Lorazepam with a starting dose of 1–2 mg, dopaminergic agents like bromocriptine (from 2.5 mg two to three times a day to a total daily dose of 45 mg if needed), and amantadine (200–400 mg/day) are useful while cases with extreme temperatures, hypermetabolism, and rigidity need dantrolene sodium. Rapid reversal of symptoms occurs with dantrolene but symptoms return if stopped prematurely. Dantrolene can be administered with benzodiazepines or dopamine agonists but never with calcium channel blockers as cardiovascular collapse can occur. Electroconvulsive therapy can be effective if symptoms are refractory to supportive therapy and pharmacotherapy

For serotonin syndrome, in addition to the discontinuation of the offending drugs and supportive care, cyproheptadine may be given in less severe cases and; if a response is observed, it should be continued until symptoms resolve.[20] Benzodiazepines or other 5-hydroxytryptamine 2 receptor antagonists (such as chlorpromazine or olanzapine) have been used in severe cases.

CONCLUSION

Managing TS presents a complex clinical scenario requiring tailored treatment strategies. While reducing or discontinuing DRBAs remains a cornerstone approach, the potential for irreversible TD underscores the need for vigilant management. Safer alternatives like clozapine, quetiapine, and iloperidone, with their reduced TD risk, offer viable options for patients with persistent psychotic symptoms. Addressing risk factors such as age, gender, and antipsychotic dosing disparities is crucial for optimizing treatment outcomes. Botulinum toxin and DBS play promising roles in managing specific symptoms of TS, offering targeted relief for dystonic movements that are refractory to conventional therapies. Future research should focus on elucidating effective therapeutic algorithms and advancing targeted interventions to alleviate the burden of TS effectively **(Flowchart 1)**.

Treatment pathway for tardive syndromes:[21]

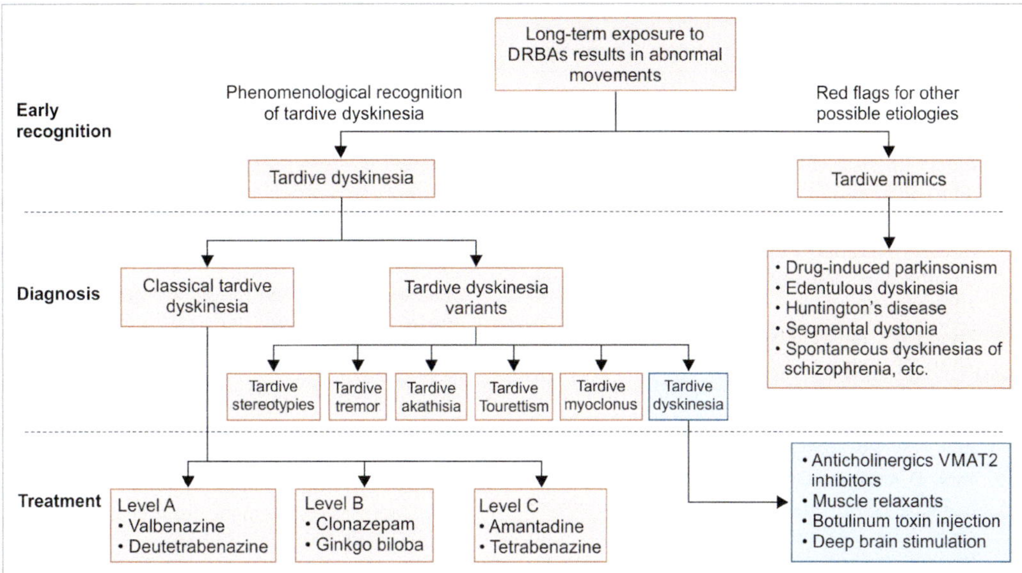

FLOWCHART 1: Early recognition and diagnosis of tardive dyskinesia (TD) and the ideal treatment pathway. Neurologists have an important role in the early recognition and differential diagnosis of TD, in particular, in recognizing movement disorder t and identifying red flags for alternative diagnosis. For the treatment of TD, neurologists should be included wherever practical, as part of the management team alongside psychiatrists, working collaboratively and with joint decision-making to determine if suppression of abnormal movements is necessary and if specific treatment is needed.

(DRBAs: dopamine receptor blocking agents; VMAT2: vesicular monoamine transporter type 2)

REFERENCES

1. Claxton KL, Chen JJ, Swope DM. Drug-induced movement disorders. J Pharm Pract. 2007;20(6): 415-29.
2. Cornett EM, Novitch M, Kaye AD, Kata V, Kaye AM. Medication-induced tardive dyskinesia: A review and update. Ochsner J. 2017;17(2):162-74.
3. Duma SR, Fung VS. Drug-induced movement disorders. Aust Prescr. 2019;42(2):56-61.
4. Strawn JR, Keck PE Jr, Caroff SN. Neuroleptic malignant syndrome. Am J Psychiatry. 2007;164(6): 870-6.
5. Bhidayasiri R, Fahn S, Weiner WJ, Gronseth GS, Sullivan KL, Zesiewicz TA; American Academy of Neurology. Evidence-based guideline: Treatment of tardive syndromes: Report of the Guideline Development Subcommittee of the American Academy of Neurology. Neurology. 2013;81(5):463-9.
6. Marder SR, Singer C, Lindenmayer JP, Tanner CM, Comella CL, Verghese C, et al. A Phase 3, 1-Year, Open-Label Trial of Valbenazine in Adults With Tardive Dyskinesia. J Clin Psychopharmacol. 2019;39(6):620-7.
7. Horiguchi J, Watanabe K, Kondo K, Iwatake A, Sakamoto H, Susuta Y, et al. Efficacy and safety of valbenazine in Japanese patients with tardive dyskinesia: A multicenter, randomized, double-blind, placebo-controlled study (J-KINECT). Psychiatry Clin Neurosci. 2022;76(11): 560-9.
8. Anderson KE, Stamler D, Davis MD, Factor SA, Hauser RA, Isojärvi J, et al. Deutetrabenazine for treatment of involuntary movements in patients with tardive dyskinesia (AIM-TD): A double-blind, randomised, placebo-controlled, phase 3 trial. Lancet Psychiatry. 2017;4(8):595-604.

9. Fernandez HH, Factor SA, Hauser RA, Jimenez-Shahed J, Ondo WG, Jarskog LF, et al. Randomized controlled trial of deutetrabenazine for tardive dyskinesia: The ARM-TD study. Neurology. 2017;88(21):2003-10.
10. Kiriakakis V, Bhatia KP, Quinn NP, Marsden CD. The natural history of tardive dystonia. A long-term follow-up study of 107 cases. Brain. 1998;121 (Pt 11):2053-66.
11. Dressler D, Oeljeschläger RO, Rüther E. Severe tardive dystonia: Treatment with continuous intrathecal baclofen administration. Mov Disord. 1997;12(4):585-7.
12. Zhang WF, Tan YL, Zhang XY, Chan RC, Wu HR, Zhou DF. Extract of Ginkgo biloba treatment for tardive dyskinesia in schizophrenia: A randomized, double-blind, placebo-controlled trial. J Clin Psychiatry. 2011;72(5):615-21.
13. Tarsy D, Kaufman D, Sethi KD, Rivner MH, Molho E, Factor S. An open-label study of botulinum toxin A for treatment of tardive dystonia. Clin Neuropharmacol. 1997;20(1):90-3.
14. Brashear A, Ambrosius WT, Eckert GJ, Siemers ER. Comparison of treatment of tardive dystonia and idiopathic cervical dystonia with botulinum toxin type A. Mov Disord. 1998;13(1):158-61.
15. Tan EK, Jankovic J. Tardive and idiopathic oromandibular dystonia: A clinical comparison. J Neurol Neurosurg Psychiatry. 2000;68(2):186-90.
16. Krause P, Kroneberg D, Gruber D, Koch K, Schneider GH, Kühn AA. Long-term effects of pallidal deep brain stimulation in tardive dystonia: A follow-up of 5-14 years. J Neurol. 2022;269(7):3563-8.
17. Damier P, Thobois S, Witjas T, Cuny E, Derost P, Raoul S, et al. Bilateral deep brain stimulation of the globus pallidus to treat tardive dyskinesia. Arch Gen Psychiatry. 2007;64(2):170-6.
18. Weetman J, Anderson IM, Gregory RP, Gill SS. Bilateral posteroventral pallidotomy for severe antipsychotic induced tardive dyskinesia and dystonia. J Neurol Neurosurg Psychiatry. 1997;63(4):554-6.
19. Kohara K, Taira T, Horisawa S, Hanada T, Kawamata T. [Bilateral pallidotomy for tardive dystonia:A case report]. No Shinkei Geka. 2017;45(11):971-6.
20. Kipps CM, Fung VS, Grattan-Smith P, de Moore GM, Morris JG. Movement disorder emergencies. Mov Disord. 2005;20(3):322-34.
21. Bhidayasiri R, Phokaewvarangkul O, Shang HF, Lim TT, Cho JW, Pal PK, et al. Tardive dyskinesia in Asia—current clinical practice and the role of neurologists in the care pathway. Front Neurol. 2024;15:1356761.

CHAPTER 7

Recognition and Management of Hyperkinetic Movement Disorders (Chorea, Myoclonus, and Tics)

Divyani Garg, Shiny Joy, Sampurna Chowdhury, Achal Kumar Srivastava

ABSTRACT

Hyperkinetic movement disorders are frequently encountered in clinical practice, the most common being tremor, dystonia, chorea, myoclonus, and tics. It is vital to recognize them as treatment varies with the phenomenology. In this chapter, we will focus on recognition and management of chorea, myoclonus, and tics. These hyperkinetic disorders can be recognized by their characteristic clinical features, but occasionally, ancillary investigations such as electrophysiological assessment are required to better delineate them. Management is directed toward the underlying etiology, which usually leads to alleviation of the movement disorder, but symptom-based treatment may be required for severe or refractory cases.

Keywords: Chorea, Huntington's disease, Tics, Myoclonus, Electrophysiology, Tetrabenazine.

INTRODUCTION

Chorea, myoclonus, and tics are hyperkinetic movement disorders which are often encountered in clinical practice. These are differentiated from each other by distinctive phenomenological features. Recognition of each disorder is important to guide symptomatic treatment. Etiology of these disorders is varied, and treatment of the underlying etiology will usually improve the movement disorder, but symptom-based treatment is frequently required, as discussed in this chapter.

CHOREA

The term "chorea" originates from the Greek word "choreia", which translates to "dance". Original descriptions of chorea date back to the Middle Ages when Europe experienced epidemics of both infectious and psychogenic chorea. It was often perceived as a curse and became known as "Saint Vitus' dance" because individuals believed that touching churches housing Saint Vitus' relics could bring about a cure.

How to Recognize Chorea?

Chorea is defined as an abnormal, involuntary, and hyperkinetic movement disorder characterized by continuous, random, irregular, and purposeless movements that flow from one body part to another.[1] When choreiform movement is severe with a violent and flinging character with predominant proximal involvement, it is called as ballism. Differentiating features of chorea from other hyperkinetic movement disorders are given

TABLE 1: Differentiating features of other hyperkinetic movements.

Myoclonus	• Brief shock like jerks last <200 ms • More stereotyped than chorea • May be rhythmic • Positive (muscle contraction) or negative (muscle inhibition) myoclonus • Stimulus sensitivity
Dystonia	• Patterned movement, twisting, or tremulous • Mirror movements • Overflow muscle activation • Sensory trick or geste antagoniste • Null point
Tics	• Recurrent stereotyped movement • Preceded by sensory tic (intense urge for movement) that is relieved by movement • Voluntary suppressibility and rebound phenomenon • Sometimes motor tics are associated with phonic tics
Tremor	• Rhythmic, oscillations occur at regular frequency • Alternating contraction of agonist and antagonist at a joint • Predictable

in **Table 1**. Characteristic clinical features of chorea phenomenology include:

- *Randomness*: Unpredictable timing, direction, distribution, and it distinguish it from dystonia and tremor.
- *Nonrhythmic* and *flowing* character and it flow from one body part to another.
- *Parakinesia*: Choreiform movements may sometimes blend with normal movements and hence can be subtle and give a semipurposeful character to the movement.
- *Velocity*: Varies, faster than dystonia, slower than myoclonus
- *Motor impersistence*: Inability for sustained motor activity. For example, "milkmaid" grip (fluctuating strength of grip) and "jack-in-the-box" phenomenon of tongue (inability to keep tongue protruded)
- *Hung-up knee-jerk reflex*: Specifically observed in Huntington's chorea, it is characterized by a delayed relaxation phase following the elicitation of the knee jerk reflex. When the patellar tendon is tapped, the extended leg remains persistently elevated due to prolonged quadriceps contraction, failing to return to its resting position immediately. This is also called as Gordon reflex phenomenon.

Flowchart 1 represents a general approach to patient with chorea.

How to Manage Chorea?

The therapeutic management of chorea will depend on underlying etiology and causal therapies are effective in cases of drug-induced chorea, as well as metabolic or endocrine-related choreas. In autoimmune choreas like Sydenham's chorea, penicillin prophylaxis may provide some benefit.[2] For genetic choreas like Huntington's disease (HD), preventive strategies are crucial, including genetic counseling for affected patients and their families. However, for most choreic syndromes encountered in clinical practice, causal therapies are often unavailable, necessitating the use of symptomatic treatments.

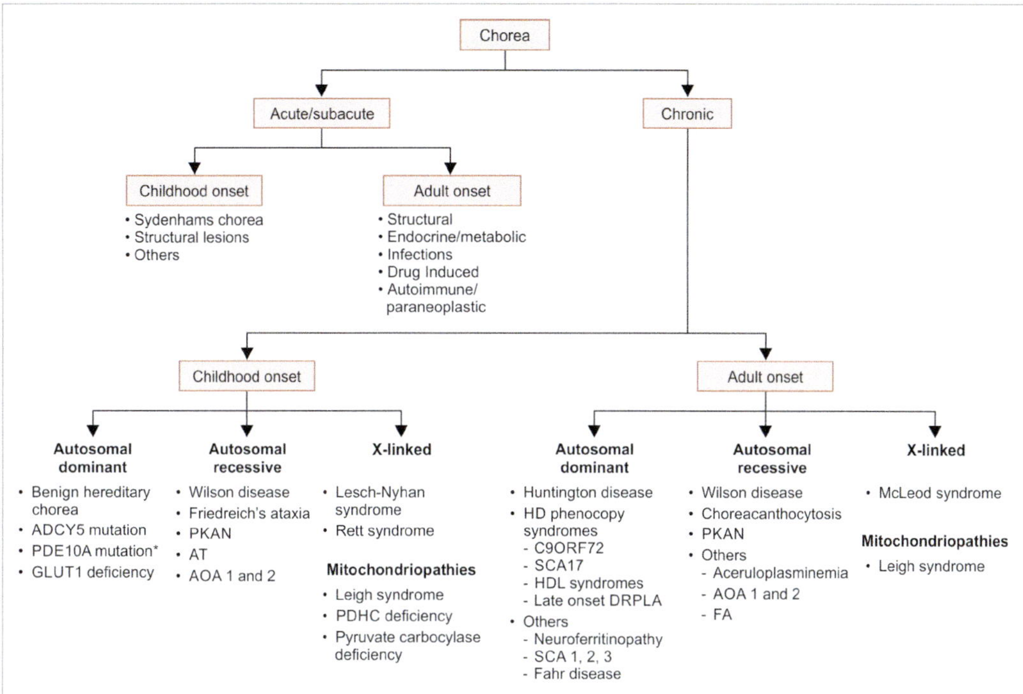

*PDE10A mutations may be autosomal dominant (more common) or autosomal recessive.

FLOWCHART 1: Approach to a patient with chorea.

Symptomatic Therapy

The mainstay of pharmacological treatment is antidopaminergic drugs, either dopamine depleting therapy or dopamine receptor (D2) blockers **(Table 2)**.

Dopamine-depleting Drugs

The major dopamine-depleting drugs include tetrabenazine (TBZ), deutetrabenazine (deuTBZ), and valbenazine. TBZ is metabolized into α-dihydrotetrabenazine (α-HTBZ) and β-dihydrotetrabenazine by the hepatic enzyme CYP2D6. According to the American Academy of Neurology (AAN) recommendations, genotyping for the same should be performed if the dosage exceeds 50 mg.[3] However, it can often be slowly incremented safely in clinical practice. α-HTBZ works by selectively inhibiting the presynaptic vesicular monoamine transporter 2 (VMAT2), which transports monoamines from the cytoplasm to synaptic vesicles, thereby allowing the degradation of presynaptic dopamine by monoamine oxidases. The first randomized controlled trial demonstrating the benefit of TBZ in HD chorea was the TETRA-HD trial. This trial showed a significant improvement in the Unified Huntington Disease Rating Scale when TBZ was administered at a titrated dose of up to 100 mg/day for 7 weeks.[4] The major differences between these drugs are outlined in **Table 2**. The advantage of dopamine-depleting drugs over D2-receptor blockers is that they do not cause tardive dyskinesia.

Dopamine Receptor Blockers

D2 receptor blocking agents include the typical and atypical neuroleptics. By convention, antichoreic activity of neuroleptics are proportionate to the receptor blocking action and by blocking D2 receptors,

TABLE 2: Pharmacological management of chorea.

Drug	Mechanism of action	Daily dose	Side effects
Dopamine-depleting drugs			
Tetrabenazine	Reversible presynaptic VMAT2 inhibitors	12.5–100 mg/day Thrice daily dose	Parkinsonism, depression, insomnia, akathisia, sedation, QT prolongation, and hypotension
Deutetrabenazine		6–48 mg Twice daily dose	Sedation and dry mouth
Valbenazine		40–80 mg Once daily dosing	Somnolence, akathisia, and dry mouth
Risperidone	D2 receptor blockers	0.5–1 mg OD/BD Maximum 10 mg daily	Sedation and parkinsonism
Olanzapine		5–10 mg daily Maximum 30 mg daily	Sedation, weight gain, and parkinsonism
Haloperidol		0.5–1 mg daily Maximum 10 mg daily	Sedation, parkinsonism, dystonia, akathisia, and hypotension
Nondopaminergic medications			
Amantadine	NMDA receptor antagonism	100 mg daily Maximum 400 mg daily	Anticholinergic side effects such as dry mouth, blurred vision, constipation; confusion, sedation, insomnia, hallucinations, livedo reticularis, orthostatic and hypotension
Anticonvulsant drugs			
Valproate	Primarily act by increasing GABA	5–20 mg/kg/day	Weight gain, drowsiness, tremor, ataxia, hyperammonemia, alopecia hepatic injury, and polycystic ovary disease
Carbamazepine	Sodium channel blocker and also potentiate action of GABA	15–20 mg/kg/day	Dizziness, unsteadiness, blurred vision, weight gain, rash, hepatotoxicity, pancreatitis, hyponatremia, bone marrow suppression, and skin reactions

inhibition of indirect pathway happens and hence, decreases chorea. Although typical neuroleptics effectively reduce chorea, their common side effects—such as sedation, acute dystonic reactions, tardive dyskinesia, and parkinsonism—make risperidone and olanzapine (atypical neuroleptics), which have antichoreic activity and a lower risk of inducing parkinsonism, preferable alternatives.[5]

Nondopaminergic Drugs

Noncompetitive N-methyl-D-aspartate (NMDA) receptor antagonist, amantadine has been found to improve chorea, coordination, and quality of life in HD patients.[6] Antiseizure medications, valproate and carbamazepine have been found to be effective in Sydenham chorea. A prospective comparative study demonstrated that in Sydenham's chorea, 83% of patients treated with carbamazepine (15–20 mg/kg/day twice daily) and/or valproic acid (20 mg/kg/day twice daily) showed improvement in chorea within 1 week, compared to those treated with haloperidol (3 mg/day twice daily).[7] Valproate is also effective in treating chorea associated with vascular hemiballism-hemichorea, post-traumatic or postanoxic chorea, and chorea related to kernicterus spectrum disorder.[2] Autoimmune chorea, including paraneoplastic (CRMP5 and ANNA1) and nonparaneoplastic (NMDA, LGI1, CASP2, GAD65, and IgLON5 antibody disease), as well as chorea associated with systemic diseases such as systemic lupus erythematosus (SLE) and antiphospholipid antibody syndrome (APLA), requires both symptomatic therapy and immunomodulation.

Surgical Therapy

Surgical treatment for chorea is rare and typically reserved for refractory cases, especially chorea paralytica, and includes deep brain stimulation (DBS), pallidotomy, and thalamotomy.

Deep Brain Stimulation

The complex basal ganglia circuitry involved in HD results in both hyperkinetic and hypokinetic movements, making treatment challenging. The loss of striatal inhibitory neurons projecting to the globus pallidus externus leads to a reduction in indirect pathway function, resulting in hyperkinetic movements. The organization of the globus pallidus internus (GPi) is such that dorsal stimulation has a prokinetic effect, while ventral stimulation has an antikinetic effect.[8]

Like other hyperkinetic disorders, such as levodopa-induced dyskinesia, the local field peak potential activity in the GPi for HD is observed in the theta/alpha band. GPi DBS is well-established for treating levodopa-induced dyskinesia in Parkinson's disease, and multiple studies have explored its efficacy in HD. Bonomo et al. conducted a literature review of 42 HD patients from 20 studies who underwent GPi DBS, finding that all patients experienced a reduction in chorea scores, with mean percentage reductions ranging from 21.4 to 73.6%.[8] The neurodegenerative nature of HD, characterized by progressive brain atrophy, cognitive decline, gait, and speech problems, makes many patients unsuitable candidates for surgery. However, patients with chorea-predominant HD may benefit the most from DBS, although careful patient selection is essential for optimal outcomes. DBS has also been used for chorea-acanthocytosis, with reports suggesting maximum benefit in those with oromandibular dystonia.[9]

Other Surgical Treatments

Case reports suggest the effectiveness of stereotactic thalamotomy and posteroventral pallidotomy for persistent vascular chorea (lasting 1 year). Additionally, some case reports indicate these procedures may be effective for chorea associated with dentatorubral-pallidoluysian atrophy, cerebral palsy, and senile chorea.[2]

Transcranial magnetic stimulation has been tried in small cohorts of patients with HD and levodopa-induced dyskinesia, showing variable success rates. However, the absence of well-defined studies and the brief duration of benefits make it a less recommended treatment option.[6]

MYOCLONUS

How to Recognize Myoclonus?

Myoclonus is a sudden, brief, and shock-like movement involving a muscle or a group of muscles, which may originate from the central or the peripheral nervous system.[10] It is characterized by its rapidity of movement. Based on body distribution, myoclonus may be focal (confined to one segment), multifocal (involving multiple noncontiguous segments), segmental (involving two contiguous segments), or generalized. Myoclonus is also classified based on neurophysiological features into cortical, cortico-subcortical, subcortical (including brainstem reticular reflex/exaggerated startle/brainstem segmental), spinal segmental, propriospinal, and peripheral myoclonus based on its anatomical origin.[11] Based on etiology, it may be epileptic or nonepileptic (physiological, essential, or symptomatic). It is crucial to identify the neurophysiological subtype to precisely delineate the management plan.[11]

Neurophysiological assessment is based on a combination of clinical evaluation and electrophysiological analysis,[12] as detailed in **Table 3**. Cortical myoclonus originates from abnormal sensorimotor cortical activity. It is clinically characterized by facial and distal limb involvement as these areas have the largest cortical representation. It is usually focal or multifocal or generalized. Examples of cortical myoclonus include corticobasal syndrome and Creutzfeldt–Jakob disease. The prototype of cortical-subcortical myoclonus is Juvenile myoclonic epilepsy and absence epilepsy. Subcortical myoclonus originates in a focal area, and spreads in a rostral and caudal direction. Peripheral myoclonus is characterized by irregular jerks occurring in the muscles innervated by a root, plexus or nerve (e.g., hemifacial spasm).

How to Manage Myoclonus?

At the initial step, the underlying etiology of myoclonus should be addressed. In some cases, myoclonus may altogether cease with this management, particularly in cases which are related to infections, drugs (e.g., phenytoin and carbamazepine), toxins, and metabolic factors (e.g., electrolyte imbalance). Usually, a combination of drugs may be needed for symptomatic management, and multiple therapeutic trials may be required.

Symptomatic treatment **(Table 4)** is based on neurophysiological categorization of myoclonus, and is discussed here.

Cortical Myoclonus

Many antiseizure medications are useful in cortical myoclonus, as they target the increased intrinsic cortical excitability in cortical myoclonus.[13] Levetiracetam, a SV2A receptor ligand, is considered to be an efficacious agent for the treatment of cortical myoclonus and has a good safety profile, and is a first-line agent for cortical myoclonus.[14] Piracetam is also found to be effective albeit in higher doses, which may lead to side effects. Brivaracetam, which also belongs to the same group with a better safety profile, has limited evidence arising from animal models, and has been effective anecdotally for Unverricht–Lundborg disease (ULD). Valproate is another agent which is widely used, especially in progressive myoclonic epilepsies, although usually as an adjunct to levetiracetam. Clonazepam has also shown some benefit albeit in high doses. Perampanel, a selective AMPA antagonist, has shown benefit in cortical myoclonus of various etiologies, including postsurgical and posthypoxic myoclonus. Other agents which have been tried in limited studies and with varying efficacy include zonisamide (Lafora body disease and ULD), lacosamide, primidone, and phenobarbitone. It is important to remember that certain antiseizure medications including phenytoin and carbamazepine worsen cortical myoclonus, and should be avoided. Very limited data exists on the usefulness of DBS surgery and low-frequency repetitive transcranial magnetic stimulation, and their current status in treatment is unclear.

Cortical–Subcortical Myoclonus

As this is usually associated with epilepsy syndromes, valproate is the first-line therapy for cortical–subcortical myoclonus. Another effective agent is lamotrigine, although it may exacerbate myoclonus in the initial period. Other agents include clonazepam, zonisamide, levetiracetam, and ethosuximide (for childhood absence epilepsy).

TABLE 3: Neurophysiological characteristics of myoclonus subtypes.

Feature	Cortical	Cortical–subcortical	Subcortical	Spinal	Peripheral	Functional
Clinical features						
Distribution	Distal upper extremities, face	Distal upper limbs, may become generalized	• BRR—generalized (flexors = extensors) with rostrocaudal progression • ES—proximal, flexors > extensors	• PS—axial, flexors > extensors, spares face • SS—focal	Rhythmic/semi-rhythmic in region of nerve, plexus or root	No fixed pattern, variable, fluctuating, distractible
Stimulus-sensitivity	Tactile/visual/proprioceptive		• ES—auditory or light stimulus to mantle area. Spontaneous jerks not prominent • BRR—spontaneous jerks prominent; reflex with stimulus over distal limbs	PS—on recumbent position at rest, rarely on tactile/auditory stimulus	None	–
Action/postural induced	+++	–	+	+	–	–
Electrophysiological features						
EMG burst duration (ms)	30–40	25–100	BRR—25–300 ES—50–100	SS—50–1,000 PS—100–5,000	50–200	Above 100
Jerk-locked back averaging EEG correlate	EEG discharges may precede EMG burst by 20–40 ms	Present	Absent	Absent In PS, BP may be seen	Absent	BP may be seen
Somatosensory evoked potential (P25/N35) response	Giant SEP	May be giant SEP	Normal	Normal	Normal	Normal
Long-latency loop reflex	Enhanced LLR1	Normal	Normal	Normal	Normal	Normal
Examples	Lance–Adams syndrome, progressive myoclonic epilepsies, progressive myoclonic ataxias, Alzheimer's disease, corticobasal syndrome, and DLB	Juvenile myoclonic epilepsy and childhood absence epilepsy	Myoclonus–Dystonia syndrome and hyperekplexia syndromes	SS—focal spinal lesions PS—idiopathic, secondary or functional	Hemifacial spasm	

(BRR: brainstem reticular reflex; EEG: electroencephalography; EMG: electromyography; LLR1: long-loop latency reflex 1; PS: propriospinal; SS: spinal segmental)

TABLE 4: Drugs useful in the treatment of myoclonus.

Drug	Mechanism of action in myoclonus	Daily dose	Side effects	Type of myoclonus drug is useful for
Antiseizure medications				
Levetiracetam	SV2A ligand	1,000–3,000 mg	Somnolence, mood issues	Cortical, cortical–subcortical [propriospinal]
Valproate	Multiple mechanisms: Increases GABA, decreases glutamate	Usual dose needed: 1,200–2,000 mg	Weight gain, tremor	Cortical–subcortical, cortical [propriospinal]
Piracetam	SV2A ligand	2.4–24 mg	Somnolence, dizziness	Cortical [propriospinal]
Zonisamide	Multiple mechanisms: Inhibits voltage-gated sodium and T-type calcium channels	Usual dose: 100–400 mg	Somnolence, dizziness, irritability, impaired concentration	Cortical, cortical–subcortical, subcortical (myoclonus–dystonia) [propriospinal]
Clonazepam	GABAergic action	Usual dose is 0.5–6 mg although higher doses (up to 18 mg) have been used	Somnolence, dependence	Cortical, subcortical (myoclonus–dystonia, opsoclonus–myoclonus), propriospinal, spinal segmental
Perampanel	Selective, noncompetitive AMPA antagonist	2–8 mg	Psychiatric issues	Cortical
Brivaracetam	SV2A ligand	50–150 mg	Somnolence	Cortical
Primidone	Barbiturate compound	500–1,500 mg	Somnolence	Cortical
Sodium oxybate	Gamma hydroxy-butyric acid salt	3–9 mg	Somnolence, respiratory depression	Cortical, subcortical (myoclonus–dystonia)
Ethosuximide	Inhibits T-type calcium channels	500–2,000 mg	Drowsiness, lethargy, headache	Cortical–subcortical (childhood absence epilepsy)
Lamotrigine	Inhibits voltage-gated sodium channels	100–600 mg	Drowsiness, diplopia, ataxia	Cortical–subcortical (JME)
Topiramate	Multiple mechanisms: Inhibits voltage-gated sodium and T-type calcium channels	100–400 mg	Somnolence, dizziness, irritability, impaired concentration	Cortical–subcortical, subcortical [opsoclonus–myoclonus]
Lacosamide	Multiple mechanisms: Enhances slow inactivation of voltage-gated sodium channels, CRMP2	100–400 mg	Diplopia, ataxia, drowsiness	Cortical

Continued

Continued

Drug	Mechanism of action in myoclonus	Daily dose	Side effects	Type of myoclonus drug is useful for
Carbamazepine	Inhibits voltage-gated sodium channels	200–800 mg	Diplopia, ataxia, drowsiness	Peripheral, [propriospinal]
Oxcarbazepine	Inhibits voltage-gated sodium channels	300–600 mg	Diplopia, ataxia, drowsiness	Peripheral, [propriospinal]
Gabapentin	Inhibits calcium influx	900–1,600 mg	Sedation	Peripheral
Other agents				
Baclofen	GABA-B agonist	10–40 mg	Sedation, lowers seizure threshold	Palatal tremor, spinal segmental
Tetrabenazine	VMAT-2 inhibitor (depleted presynaptic dopamine)	25–100 mg	Depression, parkinsonism	Palatal tremor, spinal segmental, myoclonus–dystonia
Trihexyphenidyl	Anticholinergic	2–6 mg, higher doses in children	Dry mouth, confusion, cognitive issues	Palatal tremor, spinal segmental, myoclonus–dystonia
Botulinum toxin	Blocks presynaptic acetylcholine release	As per muscle	Muscle weakness (transitory)	Palatal tremor, spinal segmental

"[ ]" indicates that only anecdotal evidence is available.

(CRMP2: collapsin response mediator protein 2; GABA: gamma amino butyric acid; SV2A: synaptic vesicle 2A; VMAT: vesicle monoamine transporter)

Subcortical Myoclonus

Myoclonus–Dystonia Syndrome

In the myoclonus-dystonia syndrome (MDS), related to SGCE and related mutations, GABAergic pathways at the level of the basal ganglia in the striato-thalamo-cortical pathway seem to play a major role, evidenced by the robust response to alcohol seen in these patients. GABAergic drugs like clonazepam are useful for myoclonus. Zonisamide has also shown some efficacy in a randomized trial.[15] Sodium oxybate, anticholinergics, and TBZ have shown anecdotal benefit.[16] DBS of the globus pallidus interna or ventralis intermediate nucleus (VIM) of the thalamus has been reported to be beneficial in a systematic review of 40 patients, with GPi demonstrating superior response in terms of dystonia,[17] and may be considered in patients who are refractory to medical management.

Opsoclonus–Myoclonus Syndrome

Opsoclonus-myoclonus syndrome (OMS) is a distinct entity which may originate from paraneoplastic, immune-mediated, or infectious causes. Treatment of the underlying etiology including immune therapy in immune-mediated causes will lead to improvement in myoclonus in most cases. Symptomatic treatment includes clonazepam, valproate, piracetam and reserpine in a few cases.

Brainstem Reticular Reflex (Nonsegmental) Myoclonus

This may respond to clonazepam or 5-hydroxytryptophan. Correction of any underlying metabolic factor such as uremia may lead to resolution of the myoclonus.

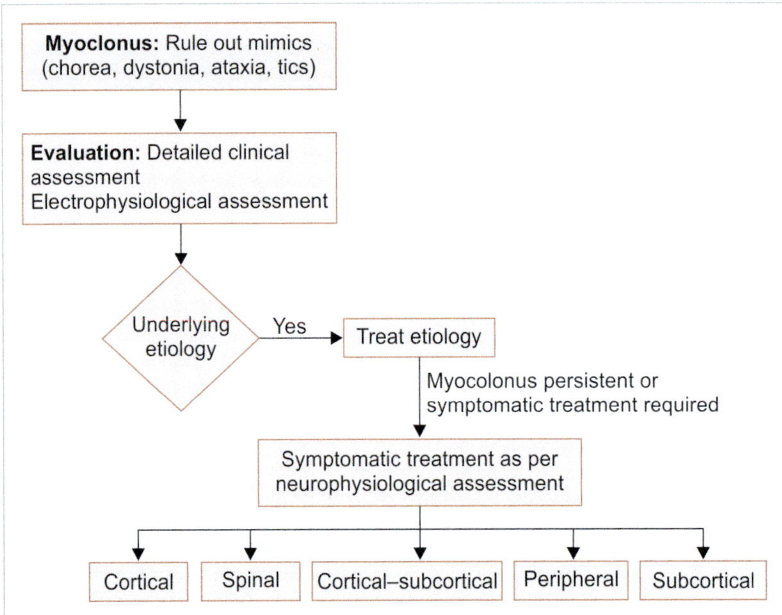

FLOWCHART 2: Treatment algorithm for myoclonus.

Brainstem Segmental Myoclonus

A wide variety of drugs have been tried in the treatment of palatal tremor with varying success. These include clonazepam, valproate, zonisamide, flunarizine, carbamazepine, piracetam, TBZ, etc.[18] Botulinum toxin is also effective in palatal tremor. In disturbing "ear clicks", surgical treatments such as tenotomy of tensor veli palatini or Eustachian tube occlusion may be offered.

Spinal Myoclonus

Propriospinal Myoclonus

Clonazepam and zonisamide have been found useful for propriospinal myoclonus, which is increasingly believed to be a functional movement disorder, although rarely, structural spinal lesions may lead to this.[19]

Spinal Segmental Myoclonus

Drugs useful in spinal segmental myoclonus include mainly clonazepam and levetiracetam in some cases, although it usually tends to be refractory to medical management. Other drugs which may occasionally be useful include topiramate, carbamazepine, trihexyphenidyl, baclofen, piracetam, and TBZ. Even botulinum toxin therapy may be useful in focal myoclonus.

Peripheral Myoclonus

Botulinum toxin therapy is very effective in the management of hemifacial spasm. Pharmacological treatment in the form of carbamazepine or oxcarbazepine is sometimes used although benefit is very limited. Surgical management with decompression of the facial nerve may be necessary in some cases **(Flowchart 2)**.

TICS

Tics are brief intermittent movements or sounds that resemble voluntary actions but appear suddenly, irregularly, often exaggerated in intensity and are repetitive and inopportune to social context.[20] They are a spectrum of neurobehavioral syndromes that lie on the cusp of psychiatry and neurology, although nowadays believed to be organic rather than purely psychiatric. Based on the Diagnostic and Statistical Manual of Mental Disorders, Fifth Edition (DSM-5), tics are defined as sudden, rapid, recurrent, nonrhythmic motor movements, or vocalizations. Tics can be either simple or complex:

- *Simple motor tics*: Eye blinking, shoulder shrugging, and extension of extremities. They usually are of short duration, i.e., milliseconds.
- *Simple vocal tics*: Throat clearing, sniffing, and grunting.
- *Complex motor tics*: Combination of simple tics such as simultaneous head turning and shoulder shrugging.
- *Complex tics*: These may appear purposeful such as imitation behavior/obscene gestures (copropraxia).

Tic disorders in turn can be classified into:

- Tourette syndrome (TS)
- Chronic persistent motor or vocal tics
- Provisional tic disorder
- Other specified and unspecified tic disorder

Table 5 summarizes the DSM-5 diagnostic criteria for tic disorders.[21]

How to Identify Tics?

Tics are relatively brief intermittent, repetitive, and stereotyped muscle contractions resulting in motor movements or production of sounds (vocal or phonic tics). They are preceded by premonitory sensations in >80% patients. This helps to differentiate tics from other brief hyperkinetic movements such as myoclonus or chorea.[22] The premonitions are usually a sensation or discomfort such as burning in the eye before eye blinking/tension in the neck, a "wound up" or tense feeling inside which is relieved by jerking of the head and may even be a generalized urge or obsessive thoughts to perform the tic which disappears after the performance of the tic, at least temporarily. Unlike most other movement disorders, tics generally persist in sleep.

Although TS patients have no cognitive deficits, based on the TIC database of 6,805 cases, only 12% had tics alone—55% TS patients had attention deficit hyperactivity disorder (ADHD).[23] Other psychological comorbidities include obsessive compulsive disorder (OCD) (27%), impulse control disorder, oppositional defiant disorder, anxiety, depression, conduct disorder, severe temper outbursts, rage attacks, and inappropriate sexual behavior **(Fig. 1)**.

TABLE 5: The Diagnostic and Statistical Manual of Mental Disorders, Fifth Edition (DSM-5) criteria for the diagnosis of various tic disorders.

Tourette syndrome (TS)	Chronic persistent motor or vocal tics	Provisional tic disorder
Both multiple motor and one or more vocal tics, at some point in the disease, not necessarily simultaneously	Single or multiple motor or vocal tics but not both	Single or multiple motor and/or vocal tics
Persisted for at least 1 year—may wax or wane	Persisted for at least 1 year—may wax or wane	Present for <1 year
Onset < 18 years	Onset < 18 years	Onset < 18 years
Other causes are excluded	Other causes are excluded	Other causes are excluded
	Criteria has never met TS	Criteria has never met TS

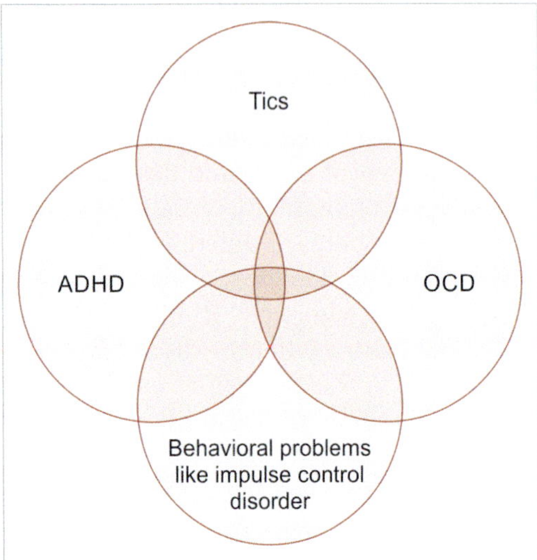

FIG. 1: Psychiatric comorbidities in tics.

(ADHD: attention deficit hyperactivity disorder; OCD: obsessive compulsive disorder)

Tourette syndrome is probably the most common cause of tics. Till date, only two genes have been identified to cause pathogenicity in tics—*SLITRK1* gene on chromosome 13 and the *histidine decarboxylase (HDC)* gene on chromosome 15.[24] However, several secondary causes have also been identified **(Box 1)**. There has been a controversy regarding immunologic mechanisms in the pathogenesis of tics and several studies have suggested exacerbation of TS symptoms to have a correlation with Group A beta-hemolytic streptococcal infection prior to the event—found to have raised antistreptolysin O (ASO) titers and presence of serum anti-neuronal antibodies. However, in a case control study of 678,862 patients, no evidence was found for a strong relationship between OCD or TS and streptococcal infections **(Flowchart 3)**.[25]

How to Manage Tics?

The most important aspect in managing tic disorder is education and awareness generation among parents, teachers, classmates and the people who regularly interact with the patient, about the disorder.[26] For a child, it is perhaps more important to advocate the best possible school environment which should include extra time/breaks to allow release of tics and alleviate stress. Therapy must be individualized as tic disorders have various manifestations and associated behavioral disorders. The various modalities of treatment which can be offered to the patient include:

- *Behavioral therapy*: The AAN recommends Comprehensive Behavioral Intervention for Tics (CBIT) over psychoeducation in reducing the severity of tics.[27]
- *Pharmacological therapy*: See **Table 6**.

BOX 1: Etiology of tics.

- Inherited: Tourette syndrome–SLITRK1 and HDC
- Inherited: Huntington's disease, primary dystonia, neurodegeneration with brain iron accumulation (NBIA), neuroacanthocytosis, Wilson's disease, tuberous sclerosis, and Duchenne muscular dystrophy
- Infections: Encephalitis, neurosyphilis, Creutzfeldt–Jakob disease, and Sydenham disease
- Drugs: Amphetamines, methylphenidate, cocaine, levodopa, carbamazepine, phenytoin, phenobarbitone, lamotrigine, antipsychotics, and other dopamine receptor blockers (tardive tics or tardive tourettism)
- Toxins: Carbon monoxide
- Developmental: Static encephalopathy of childhood with neurodegeneration in adulthood (SENDAS), mental retardation syndromes, Asperger's syndrome, and autism spectrum disorders
- Chromosomal disorders: Down's syndrome, Klinefelter's syndrome, XYY phenotype, Fragile X syndrome, citrullinemia, and Beckwith–Wiedemann syndrome
- Others: Head injury, stroke, schizophrenia, and neurodegenerative disorders

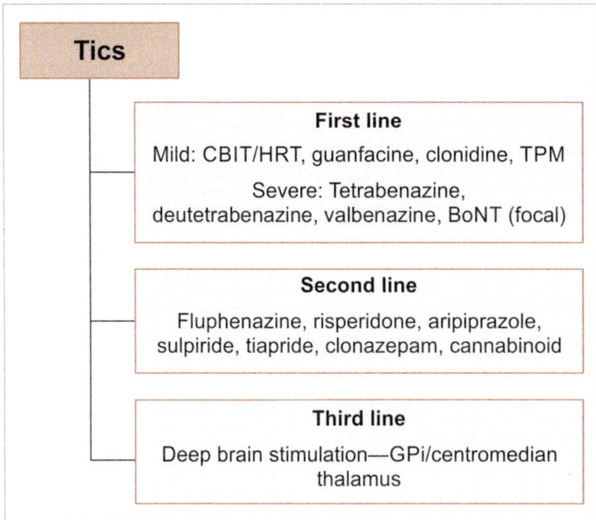

FLOWCHART 3: Management algorithm for tics.

(CBIT: Comprehensive Behavioral Intervention for Tics; GPi: globus pallidus internus; HRT: habit reversal therapy)

TABLE 6: Pharmacological management of tics.

Class of drug	Starting Dose (mg/dL)	Typical dose (mg/dL)	Side effects
Alpha-2 agonists			
Clonidine	0.025–0.05	0.1–0.3	Sedation and hypotension
Guanfacine	0.5	1.5–3	Rebound hypertension
Typical antipsychotics			
Haloperidol	0.25–0.5	1–4	EPS, sedation, and weight gain
Pimozide	0.5–1	2–8	QTc prolongation
Fluphenazine	0.5–1	1.5–10	Better tolerated than haloperidol
Atypical antipsychotics			
Risperidone	0.25–0.5	1–3	Sedation, weight gain, dyslipidemia
Ziprasidone	20	20–80	QTc prolongation and weight gain
Aripiprazole	2.5–5	10–20	Sedation and weight gain
Olanzapine	2.5–5	10–20	Sedation, weight gain, and dyslipidemia
Quetiapine	25–50	75–300	Sedation and weight gain

(EPS: extrapyramidal syndrome)

- *Botulinum toxin therapy*: Useful in treatment of focal motor tics and in some phonic tics such as coprolalia—they decrease premonitory urges as well.[28] In an open label study, mean dose was 119.9 U (range 15-273 U). Sites of injections included cervical or upper thoracic area, upper face, lower face, vocal cords, upper back and/or shoulder, scalp, forearm, leg, and rectus abdominis.

Complications included neck weakness, dysphagia, ptosis, nausea, hypophonia, fatigue, and generalized weakness, all of which were mild and transient.[29]

- *Surgical therapy*: DBS targeting several subcortical structures have been proposed but randomized trials are lacking. In an international DBS registry involving 185 patients treated with DBS targeting centromedian thalamic region (57%), anterior globus pallidus (25%), and other areas, the Yale Global Tic Severity Scale (YGTSS) mean total score improved by 45%.[30]

CONCLUSION

Hyperkinetic movement disorders such as chorea, myoclonus, and tics require identification of phenomenology for appropriate management. In tics, it is crucial to recognize and address associated psychiatric comorbidities as well. While treating the underlying etiology usually leads to resolution of the hyperkinetic movement disorder, it is also important to be abreast of symptom-based treatment to alleviate the patient's discomfort.

REFERENCES

1. Macerollo A, Martino D. What is new in tics, dystonia and chorea? Clin Med (Lond). 2016;16(4):383-9.
2. Cardoso F, Seppi K, Mair KJ, Wenning GK, Poewe W. Seminar on choreas. Lancet Neurol. 2006;5(7): 589-602.
3. Armstrong MJ, Miyasaki JM; American Academy of Neurology. Evidence-based guideline: pharmacologic treatment of chorea in Huntington disease: report of the guideline development subcommittee of the American Academy of Neurology. Neurology. 2012;79(6):597-603.
4. Frank S. Tetrabenazine as anti-chorea therapy in Huntington disease: an open-label continuation study. Huntington Study Group/TETRA-HD Investigators. BMC Neurol. 2009;9:62.
5. Coppen EM, Roos RAC. Current Pharmacological Approaches to Reduce Chorea in Huntington's Disease. Drugs. 2017;77(1):29-46.
6. Bashir H, Jankovic J. Treatment options for chorea. Expert Rev Neurother. 2018;18(1):51-63.
7. Peña J, Mora E, Cardozo J, Molina O, Montiel C. Comparison of the efficacy of carbamazepine, haloperidol and valproic acid in the treatment of children with Sydenham's chorea: clinical follow-up of 18 patients. Arq Neuropsiquiatr. 2002; 60(2-B):374-7.
8. Bonomo R, Elia AE, Bonomo G, Romito LM, Mariotti C, Devigili G, et al. Deep brain stimulation in Huntington's disease: a literature review. Neurol Sci. 2021;42(11):4447-57.
9. He W, Li C, Dong H, Shao L, Yin B, Li D, et al. Pallidus Stimulation for Chorea-Acanthocytosis: A Systematic Review and Meta-Analysis of Individual Data. J Mov Disord. 2022;15(3):197-205.
10. Caviness JN, Brown P. Myoclonus: current concepts and recent advances. Lancet Neurol. 2004;3(10):598-607.
11. Pena AB, Caviness JN. Physiology-Based Treatment of Myoclonus. Neurotherapeutics. 2020;17(4):1665-80.
12. Chen KHS, Chen R. Principles of Electrophysiological Assessments for Movement Disorders. JMD. 2020;13(1):27-38.
13. Ugawa Y, Uesaka Y, Terao Y, Yumoto M, Hnajima R, Sakai K. Pathophysiology of sensorimotor cortex in cortical myoclonus. Clin Neurosci. 1995;3(4):198-202.
14. Caviness JN. Treatment of Myoclonus. Neurotherapeutics. 2014;11(1):188-200.
15. Hainque E, Vidailhet M, Cozic N, Charbonnier-Beaupel F, Thobois S, Tranchant C, et al. A randomized, controlled, double-blind, crossover trial of zonisamide in myoclonus-dystonia. Neurology. 2016;86(18):1729-35.
16. Fearon C, Peall KJ, Vidailhet M, Fasano A. Medical management of myoclonus-dystonia and implications for underlying pathophysiology. Parkinsonism Relat Disord. 2020;77:48-56.
17. Rughani AI, Lozano AM. Surgical treatment of myoclonus dystonia syndrome. Mov Disord. 2013;28(3):282-7.
18. Bhattacharjee S. Palatal Tremor–Pathophysiology, Clinical Features, Investigations, Management and Future Challenges. Tremor Other Hyperkinet Mov (N Y). 2020;10:40.

19. van der Salm SMA, Erro R, Cordivari C, Edwards MJ, Koelman JH, van den Ende T, et al. Propriospinal myoclonus. Neurology. 2014;83(20):1862-70.
20. Ganos C. Tics and Tourette's: update on pathophysiology and tic control. Curr Opin Neurol. 2016;29(4):513-8.
21. Regier DA, Kuhl EA, Kupfer DJ. The DSM-5: Classification and criteria changes. World Psychiatry. 2013;12(2):92.
22. Reese HE, Scahill L, Peterson AL, Crowe K, Woods DW, Piacentini J, et al. The premonitory urge to tic: measurement, characteristics, and correlates in older adolescents and adults. Behav Ther. 2014;45(2):177-86.
23. Freeman RD, Tourette Syndrome International Database Consortium. Tic disorders and ADHD: answers from a world-wide clinical dataset on Tourette syndrome. Eur Child Adolesc Psychiatry. 2007;16 Suppl 1:15-23.
24. Lin WD, Tsai FJ, Chou IC. Current understanding of the genetics of Tourette syndrome. Biomed J. 2022;45(2):271-9.
25. Schrag A, Gilbert R, Giovannoni G, Robertson MM, Metcalfe C, Ben-Shlomo Y. Streptococcal infection, Tourette syndrome, and OCD: is there a connection? Neurology. 2009;73(16):1256-63.
26. Jankovic J. Treatment of tics associated with Tourette syndrome. J Neural Transm (Vienna). 2020;127(5):843-50.
27. Pringsheim T, Holler-Managan Y, Okun MS, ankovic J, Piacentini J, Cavanna AE, et al. Comprehensive systematic review summary: Treatment of tics in people with Tourette syndrome and chronic tic disorders. Neurology. 2019;92(19):907-15.
28. Marras C, Andrews D, Sime E, Lang AE. Botulinum toxin for simple motor tics: a randomized, double-blind, controlled clinical trial. Neurology. 2001;56(5):605-10.
29. Kwak CH, Hanna PA, Jankovic J. Botulinum toxin in the treatment of tics. Arch Neurol. 2000;57(8):1190-3.
30. Martinez-Ramirez D, Jimenez-Shahed J, Leckman JF, Porta M, Servello D, Meng FG, et al. Efficacy and Safety of Deep Brain Stimulation in Tourette Syndrome: The International Tourette Syndrome Deep Brain Stimulation Public Database and Registry. JAMA Neurol. 2018;75(3):353-9.

CHAPTER

8

Therapeutic Options in Tremor Disorders

Kartika Gulati, Sanjay Pandey

ABSTRACT

Tremor is the most common condition encountered in movement disorder clinics. The newer classification system proposed by the International Parkinson and Movement Disorder Society focuses on clinical features, phenomenology, and etiology. In addition to the clinical examination, neuroimaging, and biomarker analysis can also help to identify the tremor phenomenology. Treatment strategies for tremors include pharmacotherapy, botulinum toxin injections, and surgical interventions such as lesional surgeries and neuromodulation (deep brain stimulation). This comprehensive review provides a descriptive commentary on the new tremor classification. It sheds light on the evolving landscape of tremor management, especially essential tremor syndrome and dystonic tremor, and excludes the treatment of parkinsonian tremors, for a more focused discussion.

Keywords: Tremor, Essential tremor, Dystonic tremor, Treatment.

INTRODUCTION

Tremor is the most common presentation in movement disorder clinics. The etiology and phenomenology of tremor syndromes are heterogenous. This narrative review aims to provide a comprehensive overview of the newer classification for tremor syndromes and to explore the heterogeneous etiology and phenomenology of tremor syndromes commonly seen in movement disorder clinics. We also aim to review the current diagnostic strategies for classifying tremor syndromes, including the role of surface electromyography (EMG), neuroimaging, and biomarkers. Here, we have discussed the treatment modalities for tremor syndromes, focusing particularly on essential tremor and dystonic tremor, as well as addressing rarer syndromes such as Holme's tremor. We have not included the treatment of parkinsonian tremors. These aims outline the scope of our narrative review, highlighting the focus on the classification, diagnosis, and treatment of various tremor syndromes, while excluding the treatment of parkinsonian tremors for a more targeted discussion.

DEFINITION AND CLASSIFICATION

Tremor is an involuntary, rhythmic, and oscillatory movement involving one or several body parts.[1,2] The International Parkinson and Movement Disorder Society 2018 consensus guidelines on tremor classification give a biaxial approach.[1] Axis-I comprises history, clinical examination, and tremor characteristics.[1] Tremor characteristics include region of distribution (focal, segmental, hemi-tremor, or generalized), activation conditions (at rest or during action) and tremor frequency.[3] In addition to the history taking and clinical examination, certain investigations like surface EMG, structural neuroimaging, dopamine and serotonin transporter scans, and serum/tissue biomarkers can be helpful.[4] After determining the phenomenology of tremor in Axis-I, the next step is to determine the tremor etiology in Axis-II.[1] Tremor etiology is divided into genetically defined, acquired or idiopathic.

Rest tremor is present when the involved extremity is completely supported against gravity and subsides upon performing any action. Rest tremor in Parkinson's disease (PD) is a "pill-rolling" tremor of 4–6 Hz, involving one upper limb distally and asymmetrically.[5] There can be an associated and more troublesome postural/kinetic tremor, which can be of the same frequency as that of the rest tremor, and may emerge after several seconds of attaining a posture (re-emergent tremor).[5] Suppression of rest tremor upon initiating voluntary movements of the affected body part is a pointer toward PD.[6] Rest tremor can also occur as a component of essential tremor (ET) syndrome and dystonic syndrome. Other etiologies of rest tremor include atypical parkinsonism like multiple system atrophy, cortico-basal syndrome, progressive supranuclear palsy, vascular parkinsonism, and drug-induced parkinsonism.

Action tremor is when tremor becomes more obvious while performing an action and is divided into postural, kinetic, or isometric tremor.[1]

Essential tremor is one of the most common causes of action tremors. Essential tremor is defined as an isolated action tremor syndrome of bilateral upper limbs, of at least 3 years' duration, with or without tremor in other locations (e.g., head, voice, or lower limbs).[1] There is absence of other neurological signs, such as dystonia, ataxia, or parkinsonism.[1] Tremor frequency in ET ranges between 4 and 12 Hz. A positive family history and improvement with small doses of alcohol may be seen but may not be consistently present. In the recent tremor classification, definitions of ET and ET plus have been refined.[1]

Essential tremor plus is diagnosed when there is the presence of neurological signs of uncertain significance ("soft neurological signs") such as impaired tandem gait, questionable dystonic posturing, memory impairment, or other mild neurological signs of unknown significance, in addition to the presence of ET. Following this classification, many centers have reclassified their patients of ET syndrome and concluded that ET plus outnumbers the ET patients.[7]

During their course, patients with ET may develop other signs and evolve into a combined tremor syndrome. Some patients of isolated segmental postural or kinetic tremor syndromes may later develop focal or segmental dystonia that may be idiopathic or gene-related such as *ANO3*.[8] Some ET plus patients may also have rest tremor, and it may be difficult to distinguish them from the rest tremor of PD. However, the rest tremor of PD persists while walking, and the presence of rest tremor in the legs is rarely seen in ET patients.[9]

Enhanced physiological tremor (EPT) is an 8–12 Hz bilateral upper limb action tremor, caused by enhancement of the normal mechanical reflex. It is precipitated by conditions such as exercise, fatigue, stress, excess caffeine consumption, and hypermetabolic states like hyperthyroidism.[1] Surface EMG helps in differentiating ET from EPT as the accelerometer peak in EPT decreases upon weight loading due to its mechanical component, compared to no effect on the central oscillators of ET.[4]

Primary orthostatic tremor is a high frequency (13–18 Hz), low amplitude, isolated tremor syndrome that occurs when the patient stands up and subsides immediately after sitting or lying down. Electrophysiology shows a highly coherent tremor among the affected body parts, which is a unique feature of this tremor. An audible rhythm called the "helicopter sign" may be detected by auscultating the lower limb with a stethoscope or by listening to the surface EMG.[10,11]

Dystonic tremor is when the tremor is present in a body part that is affected by dystonia.[12] On the contrary, if dystonia and tremor are found in different body parts, this is called tremor associated with dystonia (e.g., tremor in bilateral upper limbs in a patient with cervical dystonia). While assessing focal tremor syndromes of the upper limbs or head or voice, it may be difficult to determine whether the underlying phenomenology is dystonia or essential tremor.[13] Presence of sensory tricks (geste antagoniste) and null point are clues toward dystonic tremor.[14,15] Dystonic tremors are jerky, variable, and there is often a flurry of tremors with certain postures.[16] There may be associated neck pain and hypertrophy of neck muscles in dystonic head tremor.[16]

Intention tremor syndromes comprise a low frequency (<5 Hz) tremor that worsens/occurs only upon approaching the target. A common condition presenting with intention and action tremor syndromes is tremor in spinocerebellar ataxia (SCA). SCA12 is the most prevalent spinocerebellar ataxia in Northern India.[17] With the use of genetic testing, many patients who were earlier misdiagnosed with ET syndrome are now reported to be SCA12. However, tremor in SCA12 is reported to have slower frequency and more proximal involvement as compared to ET.[17]

Holme's tremor is a low frequency (3–4 Hz), high amplitude, and jerky tremor that is present at rest, aggravates on posture, and further worsens on the action.[18] Unilateral or asymmetric involvement of the proximal upper limb is seen. There may be associated neurological abnormalities—hemiparesis, ataxia, sensory loss, and dystonia.[18]

Functional tremor is not a diagnosis of exclusion but rather it should be considered when features such as distractibility, variability, suggestibility, frequency entrainment, or antagonistic muscle coactivation are present.[19]

INVESTIGATIONS

Investigations of tremor syndromes are broadly divided into electrophysiology (surface EMG), genetic testing, and structural and receptor imaging. Surface EMG adds to the clinician's assessment of tremor phenomenology and expands the Axis-I of tremor classification.[1] The postural tremor in patients with ET syndromes, parkinsonian tremor and dystonic tremor may be difficult to distinguish in certain instances.[20,21] Surface EMG reveals tremor characteristics, whether the tremor bursts are alternating as in parkinsonian tremor, synchronous or alternating as in ET syndrome or synchronous bursts with co-contraction and variability as in dystonic tremor.[22] Tremor frequency of orthostatic tremor and Holme's tremor need to be confirmed with surface EMG.[23] Presence of distractibility, entrainment, and increase in tremor amplitude upon weight loading are indicators of functional tremor.[24] Dihydroxyphenylalanine (DOPA)-positron emission tomography (PET) scan can be helpful in differentiating ET patients from PD when clinical assessment alone does not suffice.[22] Axis-II of the classification explores the etiology of tremor syndromes, and genetic testing is essential when establishing genetically defined cases of tremor syndrome such as spinocerebellar ataxia (tremor-ataxia syndrome) or *ANO3* (dystonic tremor).[1,22]

TREATMENT OF TREMOR SYNDROMES

Therapeutic options for essential tremor and dystonic tremor shall be discussed here in detail including the pharmacological management, botulinum toxin, and surgical options. This will be followed by a brief discussion on treatment of the less common tremor syndromes including tremor in spinocerebellar ataxias and Holme's tremor. Treatment of tremor associated with parkinsonism needs a more detailed discussion and is beyond the scope of this chapter.

Essential Tremor

Therapeutic options for essential tremor are divided into pharmacological treatment, botulinum toxin, and surgical therapies.[25] The MDS review on treatment of ET, recommended propranolol, primidone, and topiramate as clinically useful.[26] Whereas, alprazolam and botulinum toxin type A were considered possibly useful.[26] Therapeutic options are chosen based on the severity of tremor and the region of involvement (limb or axial tremor).

Pharmacotherapy is chosen for limb tremor in ET syndromes if the tremor is interfering with daily activities. The first line of drugs includes propranolol and primidone. A combination of these two drugs can also be used as it has better efficacy than either drug alone.[27]

Propranolol was studied in multiple level-I studies and improvement in limb tremor was noted in all the included studies.[28-31] Improvement was observed in various outcome measures including clinical rating scales of severity, and functional measures of improvement.[28-31] However, the responder rate varied from 50 to 70%.[26] Propranolol formulations include both short-acting and long-acting preparations.[26] Short-acting propranolol is started at 10 mg twice/thrice daily and then increased to 20–30 mg thrice daily dose, with a maintenance dose of 10–320 mg/day. Long-acting propranolol is given 60–80 mg once a day, with a maintenance dose of 60–320 mg/day. The short-acting formulation is proven to be more efficacious when compared to the long-acting one.[25] Factors predicting a favorable response with propranolol include younger subjects, shorter disease duration, lower tremor frequency, and higher tremor amplitude at the time of treatment initiation.[32] Propranolol is generally well tolerated by patients, but it should be avoided in COPD, bronchial asthma patients, and diabetes. Bradycardia and bronchospasm are among the most common adverse events of propranolol, reported in studies.[28-31] Cardio-selective β-blockers like metoprolol are also found to be effective in patients having hypotension and bradycardia with propranolol.[26]

Primidone is started with 25 mg or 12.5 mg once a day and increased to 50–100 mg thrice a day. Patients may report early side effects with primidone in the form of nausea, unsteadiness, and sedation.[33] However, starting treatment with a low dose and gradual escalation decreases these side effects. Primidone has the advantage of reducing tremor earlier than propranolol once treatment is started.[25] Despite their widespread use, these two drugs are effective in reducing the tremor in only half of the patients.[26] Tremor severity can be assessed using the TETRAS scale on follow-up in addition to the patient's subjective rating of functional improvement. For upper limb tremor, both propranolol and primidone were considered efficacious (efficacy recommendation) with an acceptable risk, but the safety recommendation of primidone includes specialized monitoring due to its side-effect profile and potential high discontinuation rates.[26] Voice and head tremor do not respond to propranolol and primidone.[25]

Topiramate is a second-line drug that may prove efficacious as an add-on drug.[26] For upper limb tremor, topiramate was considered efficacious (efficacy recommendation) for daily doses higher than 200 mg with an acceptable risk without specialized monitoring (safety recommendation).

Alprazolam was considered likely efficacious (efficacy recommendation) for upper limb tremor, with an acceptable risk with specialized monitoring (safety recommendation) due to its side effect of somnolence and likely risk of dependence.[26]

Botulinum toxin is considered for patients with limb tremors who do not respond to pharmacotherapy.[34] Three placebo-controlled studies evaluated the effect of botulinum toxin on ET refractory to pharmacotherapy.[34-36] Two of these studies reported improvement in the tremor rating scales for upper limb tremor (especially the postural component of tremor), but not in the functional status.[34,36] Subjects also reported hand weakness, which was dose dependent.[34,36] Individualized selection of muscles after analyzing the tremor characteristics may reduce unwanted side effects.[34] For upper limb tremor, botulinum toxin type A was considered likely efficacious (efficacy recommendation) attributed to conflicting results and with an acceptable risk with specialized monitoring (safety recommendation).[26] Patients with head tremor were injected in splenius capitis and sternocleidomastoid muscles, but did not show improvement.[35] However, in a recent multicenter, randomized trial, botulinum toxin or placebo was injected under electromyographic guidance into each splenius capitis muscle and the effect was measured on the Clinical Global Impression of Change (CGI-C) scale.[37] The improvement in the subset of patients who received botulinum toxin was statistically significant compared with placebo at 18 weeks (31 vs. 9%, $p = 0.009$).[37] However, half of the patients subjected to botulinum toxin developed adverse effects such as head and neck pain, posterior cervical weakness, and dysphagia.[37] Patients report good subjective improvement in voice tremor after botulinum toxin injection (up to 65%).[38] Patients should be counseled for its side effects before administration, and these include neck weakness, dysphagia, headache, and breathy voice in a few patients.[39]

Surgical treatment options are considered when ET is refractory to pharmacotherapy and botulinum toxin, and severe enough to interfere with activities of daily living.[26] Surgical interventions can be divided into lesional surgeries and neuromodulation techniques.[26]

Lesional surgeries include radiofrequency thalamotomy, γ-knife radio-induced thalamotomy, and magnetic resonance-guided focused ultrasound (MRgFUS).

Unilateral radiofrequency thalamotomy was considered likely efficacious (efficacy recommendation) with an acceptable risk with specialized monitoring (safety recommendation), for upper limb tremor.[26] Studies showed improvement in functional scores and tremor severity of patients subjected to radiofrequency thalamotomy.[40,41] Adverse events are more severe with bilateral procedures, and include permanent dysarthria, disequilibrium, and perioral numbness.[42]

MRI-guided focused ultrasound (MRgFUS) thalamotomy was the Food and Drug Administration (FDA)-approved as a therapeutic option for tremor in 2016.[26] For upper limb tremor, unilateral MRI-guided focused ultrasound thalamotomy was considered likely efficacious (efficacy recommendation) with an acceptable risk with specialized monitoring (safety recommendation).[26] MRgFUS uses high-intensity focused ultrasound and is reported to produce significant improvement in hand tremor with comparable efficacy to deep brain stimulation targeting ventral intermediate (VIM) nucleus of the thalamus, and maintained benefits at 2 years follow-up.[43] The most frequent adverse events in the thalamotomy group were paresthesias, and gait impairment, whereas bilateral procedures resulted in cognitive impairment, gait, and speech disturbances.[26] Historically, there has been a fear of bilateral thalamotomies as the rates of speech disturbances approached 25%, but, as of now, with the help of precise MRI monitoring, bilateral staged thalamotomy may be safe and feasible for ET using MRgFUS lesioning.[44] A large multicenter trial was just completed in 50 subjects where the VIM thalamotomies were staged by at least 9 months, and the results are currently under review with the FDA.[44]

Deep brain stimulation (DBS) surgery of the VIM nucleus of the thalamus is considered in subjects with medication refractory and functionally disabling tremor, and has proven effective in the short term (6–12 months postoperatively).[26,45] It has been reported that patients may need an increase in stimulation parameters after several months, due to the development of tolerance.[45] There are also reports that DBS of the posterior subthalamic area (PSA) may prove efficacious as tolerance does not develop following PSA stimulation even up to 3–5 years, unlike VIM-DBS.[45] For upper limb tremor, unilateral VIM-DBS is considered likely efficacious (efficacy recommendation) with an acceptable risk with specialized monitoring (safety recommendation).[26] There are three major stimulation-induced side-effects, which could be possibly overcome with reprogramming.

These include loss of tremor suppression due to tolerance in the chronic course of stimulation (i.e., habituation), gait disturbance in bilateral procedures, and dysarthria.[43] In general, neuromodulation of the subthalamic area (STA) offers similar degrees of tremor suppression compared to VIM-DBS while possibly requiring less stimulation energy.[43] However, STA-DBS may have a higher chance of eliciting stimulation-induced ataxia that can be equally disabling for the patient.[43] A randomized parallel level-I study compared VIM-DBS with thalamotomy in ET patients with severe upper limb tremor.[41] At 24 weeks, there was a greater improvement in tremor severity in patients who underwent VIM-DBS compared to those who had thalamotomy done.[41] Adverse events were more frequent in the thalamotomy group.[41] Closed-loop DBS for ET is also advancing rapidly with ongoing research on the optimal recording paradigm, electrophysiology biomarker, and classifier model.[43] In conclusion, the best management for ET is still a matter of discussion. The decision to select one procedure over another depends on whether the refractory tremor is an axial tremor or a limb tremor (unilateral/asymmetric or bilateral).[26] Refractory asymmetric upper limb tremors have surgical options of unilateral thalamotomy, MRgFUS thalamus, or DBS. Whereas, for axial tremors (voice or head) or bilateral limb tremors, bilateral DBS is a better option than lesional surgeries, due to the best side effect profile of DBS.[45,46]

In some cases, the treatment of ET plus may require some special considerations such as attention to the "soft neurological signs", as these may be more troublesome for the patient. Thus, treatment in addition to the conventional treatment of ET syndrome may depend on the predominant symptom like dystonia.[25] As subtle dystonic components may not be appreciated in examination alone, it should be confirmed by surface EMG. Rarely, patients with ET may develop features of PD, leading to the ET-PD overlap.[47] Such cases may benefit from a levodopa challenge test, and it should be explored as a treatment option in these patients.[47]

Dystonic Tremor

Dystonic tremor treatment is less well-studied with a paucity of controlled studies.[48] A systematic review proposed recommendations on the treatment of dystonic tremor based on the region of distribution of the tremor.[48]

Pharmacotherapy may be effective when there is a limb tremor with or without the presence of axial tremor. Studies have shown variable responses to medications and the commonly used drugs include anticholinergics (trihexyphenidyl), tetrabenazine, clonazepam, β-blockers (propranolol), and primidone. Trihexyphenidyl (at doses 4–10 mg/day) is the most commonly used drug for the treatment of dystonic tremor.[49] Propranolol has shown efficacy in improving limb tremor in idiopathic focal dystonia patients.[49] Tremor in DOPA-responsive dystonia typically responds to low doses of levodopa with improvement in the dystonic postures.[49] Clonazepam has shown efficacy in dystonic tremor patients at doses of 0.5–3 mg/day.[50] Alternatively, primary writing tremor has shown some improvement with tetrabenazine.[51] In a study of 25 patients with dystonic tremor, only 40% showed improvement with oral treatment and anticholinergics were the most useful drugs, followed by propranolol.[52]

Botulinum toxin is considered the most useful strategy in the management of axial tremors including the tremors of the head, jaw, and vocal cord and for task-specific tremors like primary writing tremor.[48] In a retrospective analysis of 118 patients of cervical dystonia with or without the presence of head tremor, the response to botulinum toxin injection was evaluated.[53] Patients with tremulous cervical dystonia had significant improvement in the Tsui scale with botulinum toxin injection as compared to those without the head tremor.[53]

Surgical therapy can be considered in patients with a severely disabling and medication-refractory dystonic tremor. Neuromodulation includes deep brain stimulation and the target sites for DBS are the VIM nucleus of the thalamus and the globus pallidus interna (GPi), depending on the predominance of tremor (VIM) or dystonic postures (GPi).[48] Bilateral procedures can be performed in cases with axial or head tremors.

Considering the potential effect on the other dystonic features, GPi is the preferred target; thalamic stimulation may be added in cases where the benefit is insufficient.[54,55]

A recent prospective study included patients of ET and dystonic tremor, who subsequently underwent MRgFUS thalamotomy and were followed up for 12 months.[56] Tremor significantly improved in both groups.[56] VIM thalamic lesion was significantly more anterior in dystonic tremor patients compared to the classical VIM coordinates used for ET, modified intra-operatively based on the clinical response.[56]

Further in this review, we explore the treatment strategies tailored for rare tremors, including those associated with spinocerebellar ataxia and Holme's tremor.

Tremor in Spinocerebellar Ataxia

In the absence of any specific guidelines, the treatment of tremor in SCAs is based on the phenomenology and associated clinical features (spasticity, rigidity, and dystonia).[21] Common drugs used to treat tremor in SCA patients are amantadine, clonazepam, trihexyphenidyl, and baclofen.[21] Tremor with a prominent postural component may benefit from propranolol, primidone, and possibly clonazepam.[17,57] Primidone use may be limited by its side effect profile of sedation and nausea.[27] Rest tremor in SCA may benefit from levodopa treatment, especially when there is the presence of parkinsonism as well.[21] The response to levodopa treatment may be so significant in some patients of SCA2 and SCA3, that they may be confused with PD.[58] Botulinum toxin may be considered for axial tremors, particularly head tremor and other forms of dystonic tremor like spasmodic dysphonia.[59]

Surgical options for spinocerebellar ataxia have been explored in the last few years, and case reports are pursuing various sites of DBS in SCA patients with tremor refractory to medications.[60,61] The most common target for tremor in SCAs is the VIM nucleus of the thalamus. DBS of the GPi has also been tried, due to its potential effect on dystonic tremors.[60] Bilateral subthalamic nucleus (STN) DBS demonstrated long-term efficacy in a case of SCA3 with levodopa-responsive parkinsonism and rest tremor.[62]

Holme's Tremor

Patients with Holme's tremor have a response rate of around 60% with levodopa.[63,64] They may respond to other dopaminergic drugs as well. Medication-refractory disabling tremor may be considered for DBS, and the target sites that have been reported in the literature include the thalamus (VIM), subthalamic nucleus, GPi, caudal zona incerta, and PSA. Patients show variable improvement in symptoms following DBS.[64] However, objective data with specific tremor rating scales was lacking in these studies.[64]

CONCLUSION

The treatment landscape of tremor syndromes is rapidly evolving. From traditional pharmacotherapy to the use of botulinum toxin and surgeries like DBS, patients now have more choices to effectively manage their symptoms and improve their quality of life. The nuanced characteristics of tremor phenomenology play a pivotal role in guiding these therapeutic decisions.

REFERENCES

1. Bhatia KP, Bain P, Bajaj N, Elble RJ, Hallett M, Louis ED, et al. Consensus Statement on the classification of tremors from the task force on tremor of the International Parkinson and Movement Disorder Society. Mov Disord. 2018;33:75-87.
2. Louis ED. Tremor. Contin Lifelong Learn Neurol. 2019;25:959-75.
3. Deuschl G, Bain P, Brin M. Consensus statement of the movement disorder society on tremor. Ad Hoc Scientific Committee. Mov Disord. 1998;13 Suppl 3:2-23.
4. Elble RJ, Deuschl G. Tremor. In: Brown WF, Bolton CF, Aminoff MJ (Eds). Neuromuscular Function and Disease: Basic, Clinical and Electrodiagnostic Aspects. Philadelphia, PA: WB Saunders; 2002. pp. 1759-79.
5. Jankovic J, Schwartz KS, Ondo W. Re-emergent tremor of Parkinson's disease. J Neurol Neurosurg Psychiatry. 1999;67:646-50.
6. Papengut F, Raethjen J, Binder A, Deuschl G. Rest tremor suppression may separate essential from parkinsonian rest tremor. Parkinsonism Relat Disord. 2013;19:693-7.
7. Prasad S, Pal PK. Reclassifying essential tremor: implications for the future of past research. Mov Disord. 2019;34:437.
8. Stamelou M, Charlesworth G, Cordivari C, Schneider SA, Kägi G, Sheerin UM, et al. The phenotypic spectrum of DYT24 due to ANO3 mutations. Mov Disord. 2014;29:928-34.
9. Louis ED, Ferreira JJ. How common is the most common adult movement disorder? Update on the worldwide prevalence of essential tremor. Mov Disord. 2010;25:534-41.
10. DeOrchis VS, Geyer HL, Herskovitz S. Teaching video neuroimages: orthostatic tremor: the helicopter sign. Neurology. 2013;80:e161.
11. Hassan A, Ahlskog JE, Matsumoto JY, Milber JM, Bower JH, Wilkinson JR. Orthostatic tremor: clinical, electrophysiologic, and treatment findings in 184 patients. Neurology. 2016;86: 458-64.
12. Pandey S, Sarma N. Tremor in dystonia. Parkinsonism Relat Disord. 2016.pii:S1353-802030078-5.
13. Albanese A, Sorbo FD. Dystonia and tremor: the clinical syndromes with isolated tremor. Tremor Other Hyperkinet Mov (N Y). 2016;6:319.
14. Cisneros E, Stebbins GT, Chen Q, Vu JP, Benadof CN, Zhang Z, et al. It's tricky: rating alleviating maneuvers in cervical dystonia. J Neurol Sci. 2020;419:117205.

15. Jankovic J, Hallett M, Okun MS, Comella CL, Fahn S. Principles and Practice of Movement Disorders, 3rd edition. Philadelphia, PA: Elsevier; 2021.
16. Sharma S, Pandey S. Approach to a tremor patient. Ann Indian AcadNeurol. 2016;19(4):433-43.
17. Kumar D, Srivastava A, Faruq M, Gundluru V. Spinocerebellar ataxia type 12: an update. Ann Mov Disord. 2019;2:48-57.
18. Holmes G. On certain tremors in organic cerebral lesions. Brain. 1904;27:327-75.
19. Thenganatt MA, Jankovic J. Psychogenic tremor: a video guide to its distinguishing features. Tremor Other Hyperkinet Mov. 2014;4:253.
20. Pandey S, Dinesh S, Rawat CS, Thelma BK. The spectrum of non-parkinsonian tremor: A Registry at a tertiary care teaching institute. Tremor Other Hyperkinet Mov (N Y). 2023;13:48.
21. Mukherjee A, Pandey S. Tremor in Spinocerebellar Ataxia: A Scoping Review. Tremor Other Hyperkinet Mov (N Y). 2024;14:31.
22. Angelini L, Terranova R, Lazzeri G, van den Berg KR, Dirkx MF, Paparella G. The role of laboratory investigations in the classification of tremors. Neurol Sci. 2023;44(12):4183-92.
23. McManis PG, Sharbrough FW. Orthostatic tremor: clinical and electrophysiologic characteristics. Muscle Nerve. 1993;16(12):1254-60.
24. Deuschl G, Köster B, Lücking CH, Scheidt C. Diagnostic and pathophysiological aspects of psychogenic tremors. Mov Disord. 1998;13: 294-302.
25. Sharma S, Pandey S. Treatment of essential tremor: current status. Postgrad Med J. 2020;96(1132):84-93.
26. Ferreira JJ, Mestre TA, Lyons KE, Benito-León J, Tan EK, Abbruzzese G, et al.; MDS Task Force on Tremor and the MDS Evidence Based Medicine Committee. MDS evidence-based review of treatments for essential tremor. Mov Disord. 2019;34(7):950-8.
27. Findley LJ, Cleeves L, Calzetti S. Primidone in essential tremor of the hands and head: a double blind controlled clinical study. J Neurol Neurosurg Psychiatry. 1985;48:911-5.
28. Koller WC. Propranolol therapy for essential tremor of the head. Neurology. 1984;34:1077-9.
29. Dupont E, Hansen HJ, Dalby MA. Treatment of benign essential tremor with propranolol. A controlled clinical trial. Acta Neurol Scand. 1973;49:75-84.
30. Tolosa ES, Loewenson RB. Essential tremor: treatment with propranolol. Neurology. 1975;25: 1041-4.
31. Cleeves L, Findley LJ. Propranolol and propranolol-LA in essential tremor: a double blind comparative study. J Neurol Neurosurg Psychiatry. 1988;51:379-84.
32. Calzetti S, Findley LJ, Perucca E, Richens A. The response of essential tremor to propranolol: evaluation of clinical variables governing its efficacy on prolonged administration. J Neurol Neurosurg Psychiatry. 1983;46:393-8.
33. Sasso E, Perucca E, Fava R, Calzetti S. Primidone in the long-term treatment of essential tremor: a prospective study with computerized quantitative analysis. Clin Neuropharmacol. 1990;13:67-76.
34. Jankovic J, Schwartz K, Clemence W, Aswad A, Mordaunt J. A randomized, double-blind, placebo-controlled study to evaluate botulinum toxin type A in essential hand tremor. Mov Disord. 1996;11:250-6.
35. Pahwa R, Busenbark K, Swanson-Hyland EF, Dubinsky RM, Hubble JP, Gray C, et al. Botulinum toxin treatment of essential head tremor. Neurology. 1995;45:822-4.
36. Brin MF, Lyons KE, Doucette J, Adler CH, Caviness JN, Comella CL, et al. A randomized, double masked, controlled trial of botulinum toxin type A in essential hand tremor. Neurology. 2001;56:1523-8.
37. Marques A, Pereira B, Simonetta-Moreau M, Castelnovo G, De Verdal M, Fluchère F, et al. Trial of botulinum toxin for isolated or essential head Tremor. N Engl J Med. 2023;389(19):1753-65.
38. Gurey LE, Sinclair CF, Blitzer A. A new paradigm for the management of essential vocal tremor with botulinum toxin. Laryngoscope. 2013;123: 2497-501.
39. Hertegård S, Granqvist S, Lindestad PA. Botulinum toxin injections for essential voice tremor. Ann Otol Rhinol Laryngol. 2000;109:204-9.
40. Zirh A, Reich SG, Dougherty PM, Lenz FA. Stereotactic thalamotomy in the treatment of essential tremor of the upper extremity: reassessment including a blinded measure of outcome. J Neurol Neurosurg Psychiatry. 1999;66:772-5.
41. Schuurman PR, Bosch DA, Bossuyt PM, Bonsel GJ, van Someren EJ, de Bie RM, et al. A comparison of continuous thalamic stimulation and thalamotomy for suppression of severe tremor. N Engl J Med. 2000;342:461-8.
42. Jankovic J, Cardoso F, Grossman RG, Hamilton WJ. Outcome after stereotactic thalamotomy for parkinsonian, essential, and other types of tremor. Neurosurgery. 1995;37:680-7.

43. Elias WJ, Lipsman N, Ondo WG, Ghanouni P, Kim YG, Lee W, et al. A randomized trial of focused ultrasound thalamotomy for essential tremor. N Engl J Med. 2016;375:730-9.
44. Elias WJ, Tan EK, Wong J, Okun MS. Advances in Treatments of Essential Tremor. Tremor Other Hyperkinet Mov (NY). 2022;12:3.
45. Pahwa R, Lyons KE, Wilkinson SB, Simpson RK Jr, Ondo WG, Tarsy D, et al. Long-Term evaluation of deep brain stimulation of the thalamus. J Neurosurg. 2006;104:506-12.
46. Huss DS, Dallapiazza RF, Shah BB, Harrison MB, Diamond J, Elias WJ. Functional assessment and quality of life in essential tremor with bilateral or unilateral DBS and focused ultrasound thalamotomy. Mov Disord. 2015;30:1937-43.
47. Lenka A, Pandey S. Essential tremor: five new things. Neurology: Clin Pract. 2022;12(2):183-6.
48. Fasano A, Bove F, Lang AE. The treatment of dystonic tremor: a systematic review. J Neurol Neurosurg Psychiatry. 2014;85(7):759-69.
49. Hokendorf H. Combination therapy of extra-pyramidal disease with trihexyphenidyl and L-dopa: an electromyographic study with specific reference to tremor. J Int Med Res. 1979;7:19-28.
50. Davis TL, Charles PD, Burns RS. Clonazepam-sensitive intermittent dystonic tremor. Southern Med J. 1995;88(10):1069-71.
51. Rosenbaum F, Jankovic J. Focal task-specific tremor and dystonia: categorization of occupational movement disorders. Neurology. 1988;38(4):522-7.
52. Schwingenschuh P, Ruge D, Edwards MJ, Terranova C, Katschnig P, Carrillo F, et al. Distinguishing SWEDDs patients with asymmetric resting tremor from Parkinson's disease: a clinical and electrophysiological study. Movement disorders. 2010;25(5):560-9.
53. Godeiro-Junior C, Felicio AC, Aguiar PC, Borges V, Silva S, Ferraz HB. Head tremor in patients with cervical dystonia: different outcome? Arq neuro-psiquiatria. 2008;66:805-8.
54. Hedera P, Phibbs FT, Dolhun R, Charles PD, Konrad PE, Neimat JS, et al. Surgical targets for dystonic tremor: considerations between the globus pallidus and ventral intermediate thalamic nucleus. Parkinsonism Relat Disord. 2013;19:684-6.
55. Morishita T, Foote KD, Haq IU, Zeilman P, Jacobson CE, Okun MS. Should we consider Vim thalamic deep brain stimulation for select cases of severe refractory dystonic tremor. Stereotact Funct Neurosurg. 2010;88:98-104.
56. Golfrè Andreasi N, Braccia A, Levi V, Rinaldo S, Ghielmetti F, Cilia R, et al. The Optimal Targeting for Focused Ultrasound Thalamotomy Differs between Dystonic and Essential Tremor: A 12-Month Prospective Pilot Study. Mov Disord Clin Pract. 2024;11(1):69-75.
57. O'Hearn E, Holmes SE, Margolis RL. Spinocerebellar ataxia type 12. Handbook Clin Neurol. 2012;103:535-47.
58. Socal MP, Emmel VE, Rieder CR, Hilbig A, Saraiva-Pereira ML, Jardim LB. Intrafamilial variability of Parkinson phenotype in SCAs: novel cases due to SCA2 and SCA3 expansions. Parkinsonism Relat Disord. 2009;15(5):374-8.
59. Ganos C, Saifee TA, Kassavetis P, Erro R, Batla A, Cordivari C, et al. Dystonic tremor and spasmodic dysphonia in spinocerebellar ataxia type 12. Mov Disord Clin Pract. 2014;1(1):79.
60. Oyama G, Thompson A, Foote KD, Limotai N, Abd-El-Barr M, Maling N, et al. Deep brain stimulation for tremor associated with underlying ataxia syndromes: a case series and discussion of issues. Tremor Other Hyperkinet Mov (N Y). 2014;4:228.
61. Pirker W, Back C, Gerschlager W, Laccone F, Alesch F. Chronic thalamic stimulation in a patient with spinocerebellar ataxia type 2. Mov Disord. 2003;18(2):222-5.
62. Kuo MC, Tai CH, Tseng SH, Wu RM. Long-term efficacy of bilateral subthalamic deep brain stimulation in the parkinsonism of SCA 3: A rare case report. EurJ Neurol. 2022;29(8):2544-7.
63. Seidel S, Kasprian G, Leutmezer F, Prayer D, Auff E. Disruption of nigrostriatal and cerebellothalamic pathways in dopamine responsive Holmes' tremor. J Neurol Neurosurg Psychiatry. 2009;80(8):921-3.
64. Mishra A, Pandey S. Clinical features, neuro-imaging, and levodopa-responsiveness in Holmes' tremor: a video-based case-series with a review of the literature. Mov Disord Clin Pract. 2022;9(6):805-15.

CHAPTER 9

Current Management of Restless Legs Syndrome and Sleep-related Movement Disorders

Samim MM, Ravi Yadav

ABSTRACT

Sleep-related movement disorders (SRMDs) comprise a spectrum of conditions characterized by repetitive movements that disrupt sleep initiation or maintenance, leading to insomnia and daytime impairment. These disorders, categorized under the International Classification of Sleep Disorders, 3rd edition (ICSD-3), include restless legs syndrome (RLS), periodic limb movement disorder (PLMD), sleep-related leg cramps, sleep-related bruxism, sleep-related rhythmic movement disorder (RMD), benign sleep myoclonus of infancy (BSMI), propriospinal myoclonus at sleep onset (PSM), SRMD due to a medical disorder, SRMD due to a medication or substance, unspecified SRMD, excessive fragmentary myoclonus (EFM), hypnagogic foot tremor (HFT), alternating leg muscle activation (ALMA), and sleep starts (hypnic jerks).

Despite the significant impact of SRMD on sleep and daytime functioning, the true prevalence remains uncertain. RLS, a key SRMD, affects 5–15% of adults, primarily in the Western populations, with clinically significant cases estimated at 2–3%. However, prevalence estimates may be inflated due to questionnaire-based assessments. In Indian populations, RLS affects 2.1–2.9% of South Indians and is more prevalent at 8.2% among North Indians.

Management of SRMD involves a multifaceted approach. Pharmacological therapies, such as alpha-2-delta ($\alpha 2\delta$) voltage-gated calcium channel ligands, dopaminergic agents, opioids, and benzodiazepines, aim to reduce or eliminate symptoms and improve daytime functioning and quality of life. Nonpharmacological treatments, including behavioral interventions and avoiding aggravating factors such as insufficient sleep and certain medications, can also be effective.

Understanding the diversity of SRMD and their management strategies is crucial for healthcare providers to promptly recognize symptoms and initiate appropriate treatment. This comprehensive approach can lead to improved sleep quality, enhanced daytime functioning, and ultimately, better quality of life for individuals affected by SRMD.

Keywords: Sleep-related movement disorders, Restless legs syndrome, Periodic limb movement disorder, Management, Treatment.

INTRODUCTION

The International Classification of Sleep Disorders, 3rd edition (ICSD-3) identifies six main categories of sleep disorders, one of which is sleep-related movement disorders (SRMD).[1] These disorders are characterized by simple, often repetitive movements that interfere with sleep or its initiation, leading to insomnia, daytime impairment, or both. Parasomnias, such as sleepwalking (somnambulism) and night terrors, involve intricate movements and actions during sleep. In cases of REM sleep behavior disorder, these movements become more complex, appearing intentional and goal-oriented. Conversely, sleep paralysis represents the other extreme, marked by an inability to move for several seconds or minutes upon falling asleep or waking up.

Sleep-related movement disorders encompass various conditions such as restless legs syndrome (RLS), periodic limb movement disorder (PLMD), sleep-related leg cramps, sleep-related bruxism, sleep-related rhythmic movement disorder (RMD), benign sleep myoclonus of infancy (BSMI), propriospinal myoclonus at sleep onset (PSM), SRMD due to a medical disorder, SRMD due to a medication or substance, unspecified SRMD, excessive fragmentary myoclonus (EFM), hypnagogic foot tremor (HFT), alternating leg muscle activation (ALMA), and sleep starts (hypnic jerks).

While the overall prevalence of SRMD is not well-defined, RLS of any severity is found in 5–15% of adults, primarily in the European and North American populations. Clinically significant RLS affects a lower percentage, estimated at 2–3%. However, prevalence estimates based solely on questionnaires may be inflated. In Indian populations, the incidence of RLS ranges from 2.1 to 2.9% in South Indian cohorts and is higher in North Indian cohorts, at 8.2%.[2] In this chapter, the current management and updates of RLS and other SRMD will be discussed.

RESTLESS LEG SYNDROME

According to the ICSD-III criteria, RLS or Willis-Ekbom disease is characterized by an urge to move the legs, often accompanied by uncomfortable and unpleasant sensations. These symptoms typically begin or worsen during periods of rest or inactivity, such as lying down or sitting, and are partially or totally relieved by movement, such as walking or stretching, at least while the activity continues. They occur predominantly in the evening or night rather than during the day. Importantly, these symptoms are not solely due to another medical or behavioral condition, such as leg cramps, positional discomfort, myalgia, venous stasis, leg edema, arthritis, or habitual foot tapping. The symptoms of RLS cause concern, distress, sleep disturbance, or impairment in mental, physical, social, occupational, educational, behavioral, or other important areas of functioning.[1]

Pathophysiology

The pathophysiology of RLS involves a range of central and peripheral nervous system abnormalities. Central nervous system (CNS) alterations include reduced central iron stores, complex dopaminergic system changes, altered circadian rhythms, and thalamic dysfunction, along with potential involvement of other neurotransmitters such as glutamate, gamma-aminobutyric acid (GABA), adenosine, and endogenous opioids. Peripheral contributions to RLS include central sensitization to A-delta fiber input and abnormalities in microvascular function, such as altered leg blood flow and peripheral hypoxia.

Risk Factors

The risk factors include both genetic (e.g., *MEIS1*, *BTBDP*, *MAP2K5/LBOXCOR1*, *PRPRD*, and *TOX3*) and nongenetic factors. While a significant proportion of patients have a family history of RLS (40–60%), suggesting a genetic component, many do not have an identifiable genetic pattern and are classified as either primary or secondary RLS. Secondary RLS is often associated with conditions such as systemic iron deficiency, renal failure, neuropathy, spinal cord pathology, pregnancy, multiple sclerosis, Parkinson's disease, and possibly essential tremor.

Treatment

Restless legs syndrome is a manageable condition that generally responds well to pharmacological treatment. Numerous therapies have been tested in randomized, controlled trials, with major drug classes including alpha-2-delta ($\alpha 2\delta$) voltage-gated calcium channel ligands, dopaminergic agents, opioids, and benzodiazepines. Choosing the appropriate therapy involves considering several factors, such as the severity of the condition, the patient's age, existing comorbidities (such as pain, depression, impulse control disorders, or anxiety), potential drug side effects, and patient preferences. The primary objectives of therapy are to reduce or eliminate RLS symptoms and improve daytime functioning, sleep quality, and overall quality of life.

The Role of Iron in Restless Legs Syndrome

Iron replacement is recommended for RLS patients with fasting serum ferritin levels ≤75 ng/mL.[3,4] Transferrin saturation (TSAT) < 20% may better indicate low iron stores in inflammatory disorders.

Assessment before Treatment

Iron status should be assessed using an early morning, fasting iron panel (serum ferritin, iron, total iron-binding capacity, and TSAT). Iron repletion for RLS has been examined in patients with and without iron deficiency anemia. It is believed that RLS may be linked to a deficit in brain iron despite normal peripheral iron levels. Studies have shown that both anemic and nonanemic patients may benefit from iron therapy, regardless of the severity of iron deficiency. However, empirical iron therapy for RLS is not recommended due to the risk of iron overload, particularly in those with undiagnosed hemochromatosis. Patients with TSAT ≥45% should not receive iron therapy. Adults with iron deficiency (serum ferritin < 30 ng/mL) should be evaluated for underlying causes, such as gastrointestinal blood loss or conditions affecting iron absorption.

Iron Supplementation and Monitoring

Iron therapy can be administered orally or intravenously. Oral iron shows gradual improvement over several months, while intravenous (IV) iron provides quicker relief, often within days, particularly in iron-deficient patients, although full effects may take up to 6 weeks. Monitoring with iron panels is crucial, with repeats every 3–4 months after starting therapy and then every 3–6 months until serum ferritin exceeds 100 ng/mL and iron saturation is above 20%, to prevent iron overload, especially in those with hemochromatosis genes. Therapy can be stopped once target levels are reached, provided no ongoing cause for iron deficiency is found.

Nonpharmacological Therapy

For patients with mild RLS, nonpharmacological treatments may provide sufficient symptom relief.[3,5] For those with more severe symptoms, incorporating nonpharmacological measures can help reduce the need for medication.

Behavioral Strategies for Managing RLS

Behavioral interventions can be effective in managing RLS symptoms, as supported by clinical experience and some smaller studies. Mental alerting activities, avoiding aggravating factors, moderate exercise, abstaining from caffeine and alcohol, and symptom relief techniques such as walking, bicycling, soaking affected limbs, leg massages, and pneumatic compression devices can all help alleviate RLS symptoms.

Avoiding Aggravating Factors

Insufficient sleep: Lack of sleep can make RLS symptoms worse. Ensuring good sleep hygiene and addressing any issues related to sleep deprivation is important. Treating other sleep disorders, such as obstructive sleep apnea (OSA), can also improve RLS symptoms.

Medication side effects: Certain drugs, including alcohol, caffeine, most antidepressants (except bupropion), antipsychotics, dopamine-blocking antiemetics like metoclopramide, and centrally-acting antihistamines such as diphenhydramine.[6,7]

Complementary and alternative therapies: Although evidence is limited, some complementary therapies such as yoga and acupuncture may help manage RLS symptoms with minimal risk.

Neurostimulation: Noninvasive neurostimulation techniques are being explored as treatment options for patients who prefer to avoid medication. One such device, tonic motor activation (TOMAC), stimulates the peroneal nerve and has received the Food and Drug Administration (FDA) approval. This device is worn externally below the knee and can be used for up to 120 minutes per day in 30-minute sessions to alleviate RLS symptoms.[8,9]

Pharmacological Therapy

Intermittent Symptoms

For patients with intermittent symptoms that are bothersome but occur less than twice a week, nonpharmacological therapies may suffice. For others, symptoms may not be frequent enough to need daily treatment but are still disabling when they do occur, such as during long flights, car rides, or theater visits. If needed, medications such as carbidopa-levodopa, benzodiazepines, or opioids (in low dose) can help. Carbidopa-levodopa is less sedating and can be taken as needed. Benzodiazepines or opioids before bed can also work, especially for those with insomnia.

Carbidopa-levodopa: Carbidopa-levodopa is an option for intermittent RLS but is used less due to augmentation risk. It offers rapid onset and good tolerability at low doses, making it a viable "on-demand" treatment for patients not needing daily medication. Studies show it improves RLS symptoms, PLMS, sleep quality, and overall quality of life compared to placebo, and it is effective in uremic RLS. Begin with carbidopa-levodopa 25 mg/100 mg, one-half or one tablet, in the evening or when symptoms occur (preferably on an empty stomach and not with high protein food). Avoid doses over 200 mg/day to prevent augmentation. Controlled-release (CR) preparations like 100 mg + 25 mg can be used at bedtime for nighttime symptoms leading to awakening. Side effects may include nausea, dizziness, or somnolence, with some experiencing symptom rebound in the early morning or second half of the night, which CR preparations may help alleviate.[3,10-12]

Benzodiazepines: Useful for mild RLS, especially in younger patients. Clonazepam, 0.5–1 mg daily, has shown effectiveness. Due to its long duration of action, it can cause side effects such as night-time unsteadiness, morning drowsiness, cognitive impairment, impotence, and worsening of sleep apnea. Because of these side effects and tolerance issues, benzodiazepines are typically reserved for patients needing intermittent therapy or as an add-on treatment for refractory RLS symptoms.

Short-acting nonbenzodiazepine receptor agonists: Zolpidem can be used occasionally, especially for RLS-related insomnia. However, it has been linked to sleepwalking and sleep-related eating disorders in RLS patients, so caution is advised.[3]

Chronic Persistent Symptoms

Symptoms of RLS occurring at least twice a week, causing moderate to severe distress and requiring daily treatment, are initially managed with gabapentinoids (pregabalin, gabapentin, and gabapentin enacarbil) over dopamine agonists (DAs) (pramipexole, ropinirole, and rotigotine) due to the latter's risk of augmentation and impulse control disorders. Gabapentinoids may also help with RLS comorbidities such as pain, anxiety, and insomnia. DAs are considered for patients at higher risk of gabapentinoid side effects, such as those with obesity or depression, but the risk of augmentation must be weighed. If initial treatment fails, switching to a drug from the other class is recommended, with levodopa, benzodiazepines, and opioids considered for intermittent use or refractory symptoms. Regular reassessment (every 6–12 months) is essential for patients on continuous therapy to monitor for side effects and complications, including augmentation.[3]

Gabapentinoids for RLS: Pregabalin, gabapentin, and gabapentin enacarbil are $\alpha 2\delta$ voltage-gated calcium channel ligands. They inhibit the presynaptic release of excitatory neurotransmitters and are effective first-line treatments for chronic persistent RLS.

Which one to select?

Selection of treatment for RLS depends on pharmacokinetics (PK), symptom patterns, and cost. Pregabalin or gabapentin is preferred for evening or nighttime symptoms, with pregabalin having straightforward PK and better efficacy data, while gabapentin is a cost-effective alternative. For all-day symptoms, gabapentin enacarbil provides 24-hour coverage with once-daily dosing. Gabapentinoids are beneficial for RLS with comorbidities such as painful peripheral neuropathy, chronic pain syndromes, or severe insomnia. They can also be useful for treating RLS in Parkinson's disease patients receiving dopaminergic therapy or those with partial response to DAs but intolerant to higher doses, as they do not cause augmentation like DAs. However, gabapentinoids may increase the risk of suicidal thoughts[13] and behaviors and have common side effects such as mental fogging, dizziness, unsteadiness, weight gain, and leg edema. Dosage adjustments are necessary for kidney dysfunction, and caution is advised when using them with CNS depressants, especially in older adults and those with respiratory disorders, due to the risk of serious respiratory difficulties. There is also a potential for misuse and abuse.

Pregabalin: Akin to gabapentin, is used as an antiseizure and neuropathic pain medication and also proves beneficial in treating RLS. In a large trial, both pregabalin (300 mg daily) and pramipexole (0.5 mg daily) showed significant improvement in RLS symptoms compared to placebo, with pregabalin exhibiting a lower rate of augmentation. The recommended starting dose is 50–75 mg/day, taken 1–2 hours before symptoms onset, with an effective dose range of 150–450 mg/day. Common side effects include dizziness, somnolence, fatigue, headache, peripheral edema, and weight gain.

Gabapentin enacarbil: A prodrug of gabapentin, is converted to gabapentin after absorption, allowing for more consistent once-daily dosing. It is particularly effective for RLS, which often worsens in the evenings. The recommended timing is around 5 PM to achieve optimal therapeutic levels at bedtime. Compared to other $\alpha 2\delta$ agonists, gabapentin enacarbil has consistent PK and is preferred for patients with daytime and nighttime symptoms. The initial dose is 600 mg in the early evening, with a lower dose of 300 mg recommended for older adults. The dose can be increased up to 1,200 mg, if necessary. Common side effects include mild-to-moderate somnolence, dizziness, and weight gain, leading to treatment discontinuation in about 10% of patients.

Gabapentin: It is not as extensively studied in RLS as gabapentin enacarbil and pregabalin, but available data and clinical experience suggest similar efficacy. Studies indicate that gabapentin, at doses of 733–1,855 mg/day, is effective for idiopathic RLS. Lower doses are effective in dialysis patients. It is recommended to start with 100–300 mg in the evening and increase slowly. The effective dose is 900–1,800 mg/day, given as a single dose (with a maximum single dose of 1,200 mg) or divided as one-third an hour before symptoms start and two-thirds before bed. For single doses >600 mg (especially above 1,200 mg), the administered dose may not correlate well with serum levels due to nonlinear kinetics, and divided dosing may aid in absorption and efficacy. Dose-related side effects include somnolence, dizziness, and ataxia, minimized by slow titration. However, it is important to note that gabapentin carries risks including suicidality, respiratory depression, and potential for abuse.

Dopamine agonists for RLS: Nonergot DAs, such as pramipexole, ropinirole, and rotigotine, are preferred over levodopa due to their longer half-lives and lower risk of augmentation. The older ergot DAs (bromocriptine, cabergoline, and pergolide) are no longer recommended for RLS due to the risk of cardiac valvular disease and other fibrotic reactions. These nonergot DAs are effective at low doses and are considered first-line treatments for chronic persistent RLS in patients at higher risk for side effects from gabapentinoids. The choice of medication is often based on patient preferences regarding administration route (oral vs. transdermal), cost, and formulary considerations, as well as the presence of daytime symptoms.[3]

Administration and efficacy: The clinical effects of the three DAs are similar. Ropinirole and rotigotine should be avoided in patients with liver failure, as they are metabolized by the liver. All three are excreted through the kidneys and require caution or dose adjustments in patients with moderate to severe kidney impairment (PK, pramipexole, and others through the kidney).

Pramipexole immediate-release (IR) and ropinirole IR are oral DAs used for RLS. Pramipexole IR is initiated at 0.125 mg once daily, with increments of 0.125 mg every 2–3 days, while ropinirole IR starts at 0.25 mg once daily, with similar dose increments. Most patients require 0.5 mg or less of pramipexole and 2 mg or less of ropinirole for symptom relief, but doses up to 4 mg may be needed occasionally for ropinirole. Rotigotine, a nonergot DA available as a transdermal patch, is initiated at 1 mg/24 hours and titrated to a maximum of 3 mg/24 hours. Common side effects of DAs include nausea, lightheadedness, fatigue, nasal stuffiness, constipation, insomnia, leg edema, and mental status changes like confusion or psychosis, which are reversible upon discontinuation. Excessive daytime sleepiness, more common at higher doses, can lead to sudden, unexpected sleep attacks. DAs should be used at the minimum effective dose to control symptoms and should not exceed certain dose ranges to reduce the risk of augmentation.

Patients on continuous DA therapy are at risk for the following:

- *Impulse control disorders*: DA therapy in RLS may increase the risk of impulse control disorders such as pathologic gambling, compulsive eating and shopping, and compulsive inappropriate hypersexuality, with an estimated risk in RLS patients ranging from 6 to 17%.
- *Rebound*: RLS symptoms can recur in the early morning or late at night, either due to a short duration of action of the drug or as a manifestation of augmentation.
- *Withdrawal syndrome*: Abrupt discontinuation of DA therapy can lead to withdrawal symptoms such as anxiety,

panic attacks, depression, sweating, nausea, pain, fatigue, dizziness, and drug craving, which may persist for many months.
- Augmentation

How long to treat: RLS is typically a lifelong condition, but the optimal and safe duration of pharmacologic therapy is not well established. Most data supporting efficacy are based on short-term (≤12-week) trials, with fewer long-term studies supporting 6–12 months of therapy with either a DA or gabapentin enacarbil. The most common issues with long-term therapy are loss of efficacy and augmentation.

Augmentation in RLS

Augmentation, a major complication of long-term dopaminergic therapy for RLS, refers to a paradoxical worsening of RLS symptoms with increasing medication doses. This can include earlier onset, increased intensity, shorter duration of drug action, or spread of symptoms to new body parts such as the trunk and arms.[14]

Identification: Augmentation should be considered if there is a sustained increase in symptom severity despite treatment, or if symptoms worsen following a dose increase but improve with a reduction. Other signs include earlier symptom onset in the day, spread to new body parts, shorter duration of drug action, and specific screening questions that have been proposed to aid in diagnosis.

Differential diagnosis: Augmentation should be differentiated from end-of-dose rebound, tolerance, disease progression, and exacerbating factors. Symptom characteristics and response to dose changes can help distinguish these conditions.

Risk factors: Augmentation is more common with higher daily doses, longer use, and lower iron stores. It has been reported in patients taking levodopa and DAs, with varying rates depending on the duration of therapy and specific agent used.

Management: Management of augmentation includes reevaluating iron levels, reviewing concomitant medications, adjusting DA dosing, changing to alternative formulations, or discontinuing DAs and switching to other medications like gabapentinoids. Opioids may be considered in severe cases. Careful management is crucial to avoid severe rebound symptoms and insomnia that can occur with DA withdrawal.

Refractory Restless Legs Syndrome

Refractory RLS refers to RLS that does not respond to monotherapy with tolerable doses of a DA or $\alpha 2\delta$ ligand due to reduced efficacy, augmentation, or adverse effects.

Management

For patients with refractory symptoms, iron stores should be reevaluated, and iron replacement should be initiated if stores are low. Lifestyle practices, concomitant medications, and treatment adherence should be reviewed. Additional sleep disorders, such as OSA, should be considered, especially for patients living alone or experiencing sleep disturbances. Augmentation should be considered in patients on DA therapy, particularly those requiring high daily doses.

Pharmacologic Treatment Options

The main pharmacologic treatment options include:
- *Combination therapy*: Use a combination of agents, such as a DA, gabapentinoid, and/or a benzodiazepine.
- *Switch to opioids*: Change to a low-dose opioids.

Opioids: Opioids can be effective in treating chronic and refractory RLS, especially for patients who have not responded to other therapies. The mechanism of action is not fully understood, but an interaction between spinal opioids and dopamine receptors has been suggested.[15] Although low-potency opioids such as tramadol and codeine can be tried, most patients with refractory symptoms will require a high-potency agent such as oxycodone or methadone.[16,17]

In using opioids for RLS, it is crucial to assess patients for opioid use disorder risk, inform them about treatment expectations and risks, and consider using a written agreement. Regular follow-up is necessary to monitor effectiveness and side effects. Start with the lowest effective dose, tailor treatment to the patient, and consider longer-acting formulations to prevent symptom rebound at night.

Other drugs: Several drugs have shown potential for treating RLS based on limited studies, including carbamazepine, clonidine, and amantadine. Cannabis has been reported as beneficial in case reports but lacks systematic study. Magnesium supplementation's effectiveness for RLS is uncertain. Dipyridamole and vitamin D supplementation's effects on RLS require further research.[18,19]

Special Situations

During pregnancy and lactation, managing RLS should be personalized, considering symptom severity, comorbidities such as depression or anxiety, and patient preferences. Nonpharmacological strategies and, if necessary, iron supplementation are often effective, but severe cases may require medications like clonazepam or carbidopa-levodopa, especially if patients prefer pharmacologic treatment. For those with end-stage kidney disease, RLS management is similar to those with normal kidney function, but medication doses may need adjustment, especially for predialysis patients, as most medications are excreted by the kidneys. Monitoring iron status is crucial, and short daily hemodialysis sessions can help manage symptoms.

OTHER SLEEP-RELATED MOVEMENT DISORDER

Restless Sleep Disorder

Restless sleep disorder is characterized by sleep-related large muscle group movements, requiring video-polysomnography for diagnosis. It differs from RLS and PLMD but may coexist with iron deficiency, potentially benefiting from iron supplementation. Treatment focuses on improving sleep quality and daytime symptoms, emphasizing healthy sleep habits and iron deficiency assessment and treatment, with oral iron as first-line and IV iron for nonresponders or intolerant cases, targeting serum ferritin levels between 50 and 100 μg/L. Other interventions lack strong evidence, and short-term medication use to improve sleep quality may be considered alongside iron supplementation.

Nocturnal Muscle Cramps

Nocturnal muscle cramps are sudden, intense involuntary contractions, often in the calf or foot muscles, occurring during sleep or while in bed. They can be idiopathic or secondary to medical conditions, with risk factors including repetitive stress on leg and foot muscles, certain medications (especially inhaled long-acting beta agonists, thiazide diuretics, and potassium-sparing diuretics), sleep disorders, and chronic conditions. Symptoms involve sudden, painful tightness in the calf, foot, or thigh, typically at night, lasting seconds to minutes and often leaving muscle soreness. Evaluation is usually unnecessary unless cramps are persistent or recurrent, in which case treatable risk factors and disease mimics should be assessed. Physical examination can identify underlying causes or suggest alternative diagnoses such as RLS, periodic limb movements of sleep (PLMS), myoclonic jerks, peripheral vascular disease, peripheral neuropathy, and dystonias. Diagnosis requires a painful sensation in the leg or foot associated with involuntary muscle hardness, occurring during bed time, and relieved by stretching. Treatment includes forceful stretching for acute cramps and daily stretching exercises for prevention. If initial prevention fails, a trial of selected medical therapies (vitamin B complex, vitamin E, diltiazem, verapamil, gabapentin, pregabalin, and baclofen) is suggested. Quinine use is discouraged due to serious side effects, but tonic water may be considered for resistant cases.

Bruxism

Bruxism, characterized by repetitive clenching or grinding of the teeth and/or thrusting of the mandible during sleep, can occur in any stage of nonrapid eye movement (NREM) sleep and is most common in childhood, with prevalence decreasing with age. Risk factors include OSA, heavy alcohol use, loud snoring, caffeine intake, smoking, anxiety, highly stressful life circumstances, and certain medications such as selective serotonin reuptake inhibitors (SSRIs) and neuroleptics. Bruxism is also more frequent in patients with attention deficit hyperactivity disorder (ADHD), though the role of ADHD medications is unclear. Management often involves eliminating aggravating factors such as alcohol, drugs, and medications, and treating comorbid OSA. For symptomatic bruxism, oral devices can protect teeth and reduce grinding noise, though they do not decrease episode frequency. Refractory cases may benefit from clonidine, clonazepam, or botulinum toxin A injections.

Periodic Limb Movement Disorder

Periodic limb movements of sleep are often linked to various sleep and neurological disorders, including RLS, OSA, rapid eye movement (REM) sleep behavior disorder, narcolepsy, and Parkinson's disease. While PLMS typically become more frequent with age, they do not consistently align with symptoms or sleep disruptions. In some cases, however, they can occur frequently enough to cause excessive sleepiness or insomnia, leading to a diagnosis of PLMD. Treatment for PLMS associated with RLS focuses on managing RLS symptoms rather than the movements themselves, while treatment for PLMS linked to other sleep disorders is usually unnecessary. Limited data suggest that DAs such as pramipexole, ropinirole, and gabapentinoids such as gabapentin and pregabalin may help reduce PLMS in RLS. For suspected PLMD, a trial of DA therapy is recommended, with $\alpha 2\delta$ ligands considered if DAs cannot be used. If insomnia or sleepiness persists despite treatment, reevaluation for other causes is advised. Although drugs such as clonazepam, valproate, and selegiline have shown some benefit in small studies, more research is needed to confirm their effectiveness.

Sleep-related Rhythmic Movement Disorder

Sleep-related rhythmic movement disorder, characterized by rhythmic movements involving large muscle groups at sleep onset, such as body rocking, head rolling, and head banging (jactatio capitis nocturna), is common in early childhood as the child tries to fall asleep. These movements often include rhythmic humming or inarticulate sounds, and less commonly, body or leg rolling and leg banging. Children typically have no recollection of these movements, which usually occur at sleep onset and during NREM sleep (stages N1 and N2), but can also happen during REM sleep. These behaviors are generally developmentally normal and of more concern to caregivers. However, when these movements interfere with sleep or daytime function or cause self-harm, they are classified as sleep-related RMD. This disorder is rare in adolescents and adults and may be associated with other sleep disorders like OSA or RLS, or with affective and neurodevelopmental disorders, improving with the treatment of the underlying sleep disorder.

Benign Sleep Myoclonus of Infancy

Benign sleep myoclonus of infancy, or benign neonatal sleep myoclonus, involves brief, bilateral, and symmetric limb jerks during NREM sleep in young infants, typically starting within the first few weeks of life and resolving by 2–3 months. These benign movements can be mistaken for seizures but differ in that they occur exclusively during sleep, cease when the infant wakes, and are associated with normal neurologic development, unlike the persistent jerks seen in myoclonic seizures or severe myoclonic epilepsy syndromes of infancy.

Propriospinal Myoclonus at Sleep Onset

Propriospinal myoclonus at sleep onset is a benign condition characterized by sudden myoclonic jerks during the transition from wakefulness to sleep, and occasionally during awakenings or morning arousal. Predominantly documented in adults, these jerks, typically flexor movements originating from the trunk, may extend caudally and rostrally, sometimes being extensor, though vocalization is uncommon. Polysomnography with extended electromyography (EMG) recording of multiple myotomes shows the jerks originate in spinal innervated muscles, with simultaneous electroencephalogram (EEG) recording demonstrating a normal alpha rhythm without epileptiform discharges. While MRI of the spine is usually normal, pathology is identified in 20% of cases, particularly if PSM persists during the day, suggesting possible spinal cord pathology, though no evidence links sleep-onset PSM to structural nervous system damage.

Excessive Fragmentary Myoclonus

Excessive fragmentary myoclonus is identified by surface EMG detecting movements of the fingers, toes, or mouth during sleep, with or without visible movements. It is a polysomnographic finding often incidentally discovered and is a NREM phenomenon resembling phasic REM twitches but is less common. EFM is benign and nonprogressive, occurring independently or with other sleep issues, with no known adverse consequences, and its contribution to chronic sleep fragmentation remains uncertain.

Hypnagogic Foot Tremor and Alternating Leg Muscle Activation

Hypnagogic foot tremor is a rapid, rhythmic movement of one foot occurring at sleep onset or during light NREM sleep, observed in 8% of patients undergoing polysomnography for other reasons, and generally not associated with disrupted sleep. ALMA involves brief, alternating activation of the anterior tibialis muscles in each leg during sleep or arousals, often unnoticed by individuals. ALMA is primarily identified in patients with sleep-related breathing disorders and periodic limb movements, and may be associated with antidepressant use.

Sleep Starts (Hypnic Jerks)

Sleep starts (hypnic jerks) are common sleep-related movements characterized by sudden, brief jerks of the body or segments, often with a falling sensation, occurring at sleep onset and potentially related to factors like sleep deprivation or stimulant intake. They can be accompanied by sensory phenomena, such as a sensation of falling or other brief sensory experiences, and may lead to sleep disturbances.

WHAT NOT TO MISS?

Sleep-related epilepsy syndromes such as self-limited epilepsy with centrotemporal spikes (SeLECTS), sleep-related hypermotor epilepsy (SHE), and sleep-related temporal lobe epilepsy can be challenging to differentiate from SRMDs due to their clinical similarities, requiring consideration of timing, nature of movements, aura sensations, and neurodevelopmental or genetic factors, with some cases associated with structural lesions.

CONCLUSION

Sleep-related movement disorders encompass a diverse group of conditions, with RLS being a prototype but other disorders are also commonly encountered. It is important to consider parasomnias and sleep-related epilepsy as close differentials in specific situations. Management of these disorders includes both pharmacological and non-pharmacological therapies. Understanding these disorders better can lead to prompt recognition and appropriate treatment.

REFERENCES

1. Sateia MJ. International classification of sleep disorders-third edition: highlights and modifications. Chest. 2014;146(5):1387-94.
2. Panda S, Taly AB, Sinha S, Gururaj G, Girish N, Nagaraja D. Sleep-related disorders among a healthy population in South India. Neurol India. 2012;60(1):68-74.
3. Silber MH, Buchfuhrer MJ, Earley CJ, Koo BB, Manconi M, Winkelman JW, et al. The Management of Restless Legs Syndrome: An Updated Algorithm. Mayo Clin Proc. 2021;96(7):1921-37.
4. Allen RP, Picchietti DL, Auerbach M, Cho YW, Connor JR, Earley CJ, et al. Evidence-based and consensus clinical practice guidelines for the iron treatment of restless legs syndrome/Willis-Ekbom disease in adults and children: an IRLSSG task force report. Sleep Med. 2018;41:27-44.
5. Mitchell UH. Nondrug-related aspect of treating Ekbom disease, formerly known as restless legs syndrome. Neuropsychiatr Dis Treat. 2011;7(1):251-7.
6. Hoque R. Pharmacologically induced/exacerbated restless legs syndrome, periodic limb movements of sleep, and REM sleep behavior disorder: a worthwhile consideration. J Clin Sleep Med. 2020;16(1):13S-14S.
7. Nofzinger EA, Fasiczka A, Berman S, Thase ME. Bupropion SR reduces periodic limb movements associated with arousals from sleep in depressed patients with periodic limb movement disorder. J Clin Psychiatry. 2000;61(11):858-62.
8. Roy A, Ojile J, Kram J, Olin J, Rosenberg R, Hudson JD, et al. Long-term efficacy and safety of tonic motor activation for treatment of medication-refractory restless legs syndrome: A 24-Week Open-Label Extension Study. Sleep. 2023;46(10):zsad188.
9. Bogan RK, Roy A, Kram J, Ojile J, Rosenberg R, Hudson JD, et al. Efficacy and safety of tonic motor activation (TOMAC) for medication-refractory restless legs syndrome: a randomized clinical trial. Sleep. 2023;46(10):zsad190.
10. Read DJ, Feest TG, Nassim MA. Clonazepam: effective treatment for restless legs syndrome in uraemia. Br Med J (Clin Res Ed). 1981;283(6296):885-6.
11. Hornyak M, Berner MM, Kriston L, Riemann D. Levodopa for restless legs syndrome. Cochrane Database Syst Rev. 2011;2011(2):CD005504.
12. Collado-Seidel V, Kazenwadel J, Wetter TC, Kohnen R, Winkelmann J, Selzer R, et al. A controlled study of additional sr-L-dopa in L-dopa-responsive restless legs syndrome with late-night symptoms. Neurology. 1999;52(2):285-90.
13. Molero Y, Larsson H, D'Onofrio BM, Sharp DJ, Fazel S. Associations between gabapentinoids and suicidal behaviour, unintentional overdoses, injuries, road traffic incidents, and violent crime: population based cohort study in Sweden. BMJ. 2019;365:l2147.
14. Garcia-Borreguero D, Silber MH, Winkelman JW, Högl B, Bainbridge J, Buchfuhrer M, et al. Guidelines for the first-line treatment of restless legs syndrome/Willis-Ekbom disease, prevention and treatment of dopaminergic augmentation: a combined task force of the IRLSSG, EURLSSG, and the RLS-foundation. Sleep Med. 2016;21:1-11.
15. Trenkwalder C, Zieglgänsberger W, Ahmedzai SH, Högl B. Pain, opioids, and sleep: implications for restless legs syndrome treatment. Sleep Med. 2017;31:78-85.

16. Dowell D, Haegerich TM, Chou R. CDC Guideline for Prescribing Opioids for Chronic Pain—United States, 2016. MMWR Recomm Rep. 2016;65(1): 1-49.
17. Silber MH, Becker PM, Buchfuhrer MJ, Earley CJ, Ondo WG, Walters AS, et al. The Appropriate Use of Opioids in the Treatment of Refractory Restless Legs Syndrome. Mayo Clin Proc. 2018;93(1): 59-67.
18. Oran M, Unsal C, Albayrak Y, Tulubas F, Oguz K, Avci O, et al. Possible association between vitamin D deficiency and restless legs syndrome. Neuropsychiatr Dis Treat. 2014;10:953-8.
19. Wali S, Alsafadi S, Abaalkhail B, Ramadan I, Abulhamail B, Kousa M, et al. The Association Between Vitamin D Level and Restless Legs Syndrome: A Population-Based Case-Control Study. J Clin Sleep Med. 2018;14(4):557-64.

CHAPTER 10

The Role of Genetics in Movement Disorders

S Sidharth, Divyani Garg, Ayush Agarwal, Achal Kumar Srivastava

ABSTRACT

The field of movement disorders (MDs) has seen remarkable advancements driven by genetic research, leading to significant improvement in both diagnostics and therapeutics. These advancements are primarily due to the development and implementation of high-throughput genetic technologies and a deeper understanding of the genetic basis of these disorders. Next-generation sequencing (NGS) has revolutionized the diagnosis of MDs by enabling comprehensive analysis of the entire coding region of the genome [whole exome sequencing (WES)] or the entire genome [whole genome sequencing (WGS)]. This has allowed for the identification of novel genetic mutations and the reclassification of many MDs based on genetic profiles. The integration of genetic data with clinical phenotypes has led to the identification of genotype-phenotype correlations. This understanding may help in predicting disease progression and tailoring personalized treatment plans. These correlations have refined diagnostic criteria for various MDs, facilitating earlier, and more accurate diagnosis. Understanding the genetic underpinnings of MDs has elucidated pathogenic pathways, aiding in the development of new diagnostic markers. This includes biomarkers that can predict the response to specific treatments.

Advances in gene editing technologies, such as CRISPR-Cas9 (clustered regularly interspaced short palindromic repeats–CRISPR-associated protein 9), have enabled functional studies of genetic mutations identified in patients. These studies provide insights into the pathogenic mechanisms and potential therapeutic targets. High-throughput transcriptomic and proteomic analyses complement genetic findings by providing a comprehensive view of the molecular alterations in MDs, enhancing diagnostic precision.

Keywords: Exome, Genome, Dystonia, Parkinson's disease, Chorea.

INTRODUCTION

The field of movement disorders (MDs) has seen remarkable advancements driven by genetic research, leading to significant improvement in both diagnostics and therapeutics. These advancements are primarily due to the development and implementation of high-throughput genetic technologies and a deeper understanding of the genetic basis of these disorders. In this chapter, we assess the current role of genetics in MDs.

The advent of next-generation sequencing (NGS) technologies has revolutionized the field of genetic diagnosis, particularly in the realm of MDs **(Fig. 1)**. By enabling comprehensive analysis of the genome with

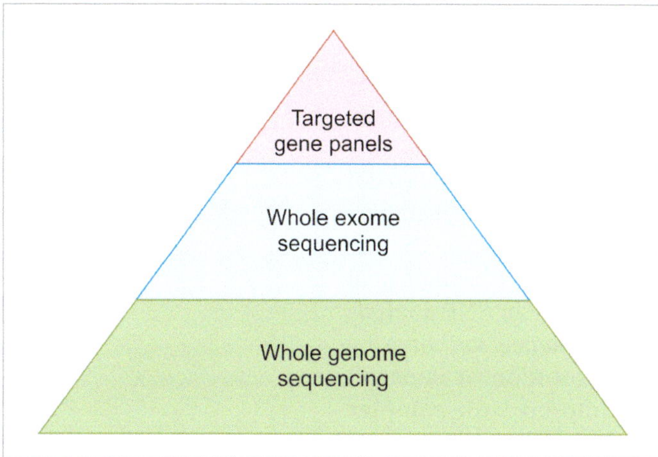

FIG. 1: The next-generation sequencing (NGS) techniques.

unprecedented speed and accuracy, NGS has expanded the scope and depth of genetic diagnostics, facilitating the identification of novel genetic variants associated with MDs and improving our understanding of their molecular underpinnings.

NEXT-GENERATION SEQUENCING TECHNOLOGIES

Whole Exome Sequencing

Whole exome sequencing (WES) focuses on sequencing the exons, which are the coding regions of the genome. Although exons constitute only about 1–2% of the human genome, they harbor approximately 85% of disease-causing mutations.[1] WES is particularly useful for identifying mutations in known genes associated with MDs and discovering new genetic variants in cases where traditional genetic testing has failed to yield a diagnosis.

Whole Genome Sequencing

Whole genome sequencing (WGS) provides a comprehensive analysis of the entire genome, including coding and noncoding regions. This approach captures a broader spectrum of genetic variations, including single nucleotide polymorphisms (SNPs), insertions, deletions, copy number variations (CNVs), and structural variants.[2] WGS is valuable for identifying noncoding mutations that may influence gene regulation and for uncovering complex genetic landscapes in patients with MDs.

Targeted Gene Panels

Targeted NGS panels focus on sequencing a predefined set of genes known to be associated with specific MDs. These panels are designed based on current knowledge of the genetic basis of the disorders.[3] Targeted panels offer a cost-effective and efficient approach for diagnosing MDs by quickly identifying pathogenic mutations in relevant genes. For example, ordering a dystonia gene panel for cases of primary dystonia.

Some other genetic techniques relevant for MDs are as follows:

- *Repeat expansion test*: Many tandem repeat diseases are associated with MDs. Current NGS techniques do not capture repeat expansions well. Repeat expansion analysis entails directed polymerase chain reaction (PCR)-based repeat length screening for most repeat disorders. However, in the case of complex, large or interrupted repeats, Southern blot may be required. Long-read sequencing now enables detected of larger expansions, such as GAA repeats (>250) in *FGF14*, accounting for late-onset cerebellar ataxia.

- *Chromosomal microarray*: Chromosomal microarray enables CNV or SNP analysis or both and has replaced karyotyping due to superior resolution. It is useful particularly in children with complex MDs with dysmorphism, intellectual disability or autism.
- *Sanger sequencing*: This is a first-generation sequencing technique which assesses small targeted regions of the genome. It is currently used for known familial variants, validating results of NGS, and rarely, to sequence a single gene.

GENETIC DIAGNOSIS OF MOVEMENT DISORDERS

Next-generation sequencing has significantly increased the diagnostic yield in patients with MDs by identifying novel mutations that were previously undetectable with traditional methods **(Fig. 2)**. For example, novel pathogenic variants in the *PRKN*, *PINK1*, and *LRRK2* genes have been discovered in patients with Parkinson's disease (PD).[4] The comprehensive nature of NGS has led to the reclassification of some MDs based on their genetic profiles. This has improved diagnostic accuracy and provided a clearer understanding of the genetic heterogeneity within these disorders.

The NGS allows for the detection of rare genetic variants that may contribute to the development of MDs. This has expanded our understanding of the genetic architecture of these disorders and has revealed the involvement of multiple genes and pathways.[5] The ability to sequence the entire genome

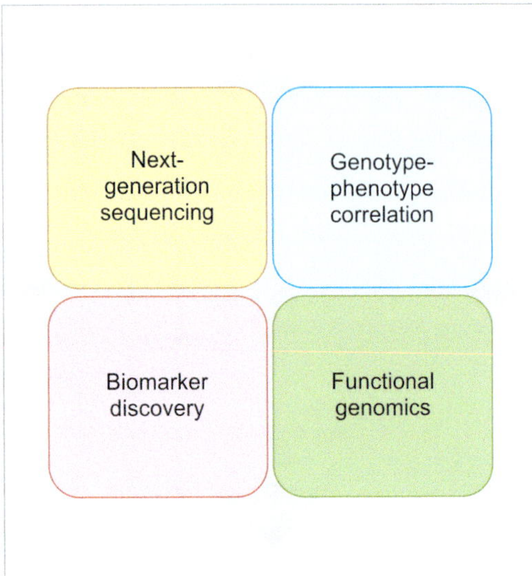

FIG. 2: Advancement in genetic diagnostics for movement disorder.

or exome provides insights into the multifactorial nature of MDs, highlighting the role of both common and rare variants in disease pathogenesis.

The NGS data facilitate the development of personalized treatment plans by identifying specific genetic mutations that may respond to targeted therapies. For example, patients with *GBA* mutations in PD may benefit from enzyme replacement therapy.[6] Genetic profiling using NGS can inform risk assessment for patients and their families, enabling early intervention and management strategies for those at increased risk of developing MDs.

The NGS has led to the discovery of new genes associated with MDs, thereby expanding the list of candidate genes for diagnostic testing. For instance, mutations in the *VPS13C* gene[7] have been linked to PD, and mutations in the *ADCY5* gene[8] have been associated with chorea. The identification of new genes provides insights into the biological pathways involved in MDs, revealing potential targets for therapeutic intervention. Phenotypic heterogeneity underscores the need for diverse patient representation in research and clinical trials. This diversity ensures that findings are applicable to a broad patient population and can help identify subgroups of patients who might respond differently to certain treatments.

Genetic counseling must address the potential variability in disease expression. Patients and their families should be informed about the possible range of symptoms and outcomes associated with their genetic disorder,[9] which can aid in setting realistic expectations and planning for the future.

GENOTYPE–PHENOTYPE CORRELATIONS

Genotype-phenotype correlation plays a pivotal role in the diagnosis and management of MDs **(Tables 1 to 4)**.[10-13] With advancements in genetic testing, especially the advent of NGS, the ability to correlate specific genetic mutations with distinct clinical presentations has vastly improved. This correlation is essential for accurate diagnosis, appropriate selection of diagnostic tests, and personalized treatment strategies. Genotype–phenotype correlations help in predicting the

TABLE 1: Key genes in monogenic dystonia.

Gene	Type of mutation	Pattern of inheritance	Clinical phenotype
TOR1A (DYT1)	GAG deletion	Autosomal dominant	Early-onset generalized dystonia, typically begins in a limb and spreads to other parts of the body
THAP1 (DYT6)	Point mutations	Autosomal dominant	Mixed dystonia with cranio-cervical involvement, speech difficulties, and variable onset
GNAL (DYT25)	Point mutations	Autosomal dominant	Adult-onset cervical dystonia, often accompanied by oromandibular dystonia
TUBB4A (DYT4)	Point mutations	Autosomal dominant	Whispering dysphonia, generalized dystonia with or without spasticity
KMT2B (DYT28)	Point mutations	Autosomal dominant	Childhood-onset generalized dystonia, often associated with developmental delay and intellectual disability
ANO3 (DYT24)	Point mutations	Autosomal dominant	Adult-onset focal or segmental dystonia, often cranio-cervical or laryngeal dystonia
GCH1 (DYT5a)	Point mutations	Autosomal dominant	Dopa-responsive dystonia, typically presents with lower limb dystonia and parkinsonism, responsive to levodopa
SPR (DYT5b)	Point mutations	Autosomal recessive	Dopa-responsive dystonia with more widespread symptoms, including spasticity and cognitive impairment
ATP1A3 (DYT12)	Point mutations	Autosomal dominant	Rapid-onset dystonia-parkinsonism, characterized by sudden onset of dystonia and parkinsonian features
PRRT2 (DYT10)	Point mutations	Autosomal dominant	Paroxysmal kinesigenic dyskinesia, brief episodes of dystonia triggered by sudden movements
PNKD (DYT8)	Point mutations	Autosomal dominant	Paroxysmal nonkinesigenic dyskinesia, episodic dystonia often triggered by stress, fatigue, or caffeine

Continued

Continued

Gene	Type of mutation	Pattern of inheritance	Clinical phenotype
SLC2A1 (DYT18)	Point mutations	Autosomal dominant	Paroxysmal exercise-induced dyskinesia, dystonia triggered by prolonged physical activity, often associated with glucose transporter 1 (GLUT1) deficiency
TAF1 (DYT3)	X-linked recessive	X-linked recessive	X-linked dystonia-parkinsonism, also known as Lubag, predominantly affects males with dystonia and parkinsonism
CACNA1A	Point mutations	Autosomal dominant	Episodic ataxia type 2 with dystonia, episodic ataxia, and dysarthria often triggered by stress or physical exertion
SGCE (DYT11)	Point mutations	Autosomal dominant with maternal imprinting	Myoclonus–dystonia, characterized by rapid, jerky movements (myoclonus) combined with dystonia

TABLE 2: Key genes in monogenetic ataxia.

Gene	Type of mutation	Pattern of inheritance	Clinical phenotype
ATXN1 (SCA1)	CAG repeat expansion	Autosomal dominant	Spinocerebellar ataxia type 1: Progressive ataxia, dysarthria, pyramidal signs
ATXN2 (SCA2)	CAG repeat expansion	Autosomal dominant	Spinocerebellar ataxia type 2: Ataxia, slow saccades, peripheral neuropathy
ATXN3 (SCA3)	CAG repeat expansion	Autosomal dominant	Spinocerebellar ataxia type 3: Ataxia, spasticity, parkinsonism
ATXN7 (SCA7)	CAG repeat expansion	Autosomal dominant	Spinocerebellar ataxia type 7: Ataxia, visual loss
ATXN8 (SCA8)	CTG repeat expansion	Autosomal dominant	Spinocerebellar ataxia type 8: Mild ataxia, dysarthria
CACNA1A (SCA6)	CAG repeat expansion	Autosomal dominant	Spinocerebellar ataxia type 6: Pure cerebellar ataxia
FXN	GAA repeat expansion	Autosomal recessive	Friedreich's ataxia: Progressive ataxia, cardiomyopathy, diabetes
TBP (SCA17)	CAG repeat expansion	Autosomal dominant	Spinocerebellar ataxia type 17: Ataxia, dementia, chorea
SYNE1	Point mutations	Autosomal recessive	Autosomal recessive cerebellar ataxia: Ataxia, myoclonus, epilepsy
POLG	Point mutations	Autosomal recessive	Ataxia, epilepsy, mitochondrial myopathy

TABLE 3: Key genes in monogenetic chorea.

Gene	Type of mutation	Pattern of inheritance	Clinical phenotype
HTT	CAG repeat expansion	Autosomal dominant	Huntington's disease: Chorea, psychiatric symptoms, cognitive decline
JPH3	CAG repeat expansion	Autosomal dominant	Huntington disease-like 2: Chorea, similar to Huntington's disease
ATN1	CAG repeat expansion	Autosomal dominant	Dentatorubral-pallidoluysian atrophy: Chorea, ataxia, myoclonus
PRNP	Octapeptide repeat	Autosomal dominant	Prion disease with chorea: Chorea, dementia
ADCY5	Point mutations	Autosomal dominant	Familial dyskinesia with facial myokymia: Chorea, myoclonus
NKX2-1	Point mutations	Autosomal dominant	Benign hereditary chorea: Childhood-onset chorea
C9ORF72	Hexanucleotide repeat	Autosomal dominant	Amyotrophic lateral sclerosis/frontotemporal dementia (ALS/FTD) with chorea: Chorea, amyotrophic lateral sclerosis or frontotemporal dementia
TITF1	Point mutations	Autosomal dominant	Brain-lung-thyroid syndrome: Chorea, pulmonary and thyroid anomalies

TABLE 4: Key genes in monogenetic parkinsonism.

Gene	Type of mutation	Pattern of inheritance	Clinical phenotype
SNCA	Point mutations, duplications	Autosomal dominant	Parkinson's disease: Early-onset PD, with tremor, rigidity, bradykinesia
LRRK2	Point mutations	Autosomal dominant	Parkinson's disease: Late-onset PD, often with a family history
PRKN	Point mutations, deletions	Autosomal recessive	Juvenile parkinsonism: Early-onset PD, often responsive to levodopa
PINK1	Point mutations	Autosomal recessive	Early-onset parkinsonism: Often presents with dystonia and hyperreflexia
DJ-1	Point mutations	Autosomal recessive	Early-onset parkinsonism: Similar to PRKN and PINK1-related parkinsonism
GBA	Point mutations	Risk factor (not directly causative)	Parkinson's disease: PD with cognitive impairment, associated with Gaucher's disease
VPS35	Point mutations	Autosomal dominant	Parkinson's disease: Late-onset PD with progressive course
ATP13A2	Point mutations	Autosomal recessive	Kufor–Rakeb syndrome: Parkinsonism, pyramidal signs, dementia
PLA2G6	Point mutations	Autosomal recessive	PARK14: Atypical parkinsonism with dystonia and pyramidal signs

clinical course, potential complications, and treatment responses in patients with MDs. These correlations are particularly useful in:

- *Diagnosis of rare disorders*: Many rare genetic disorders have overlapping clinical features. Genotype–phenotype correlation helps in differentiating these disorders based on specific genetic mutations.
- *Guiding genetic testing*: Identifying the phenotype can guide clinicians to test for specific genes, making the diagnostic process more efficient and cost-effective.
- *Predicting disease progression*: Certain genetic mutations are associated with more severe disease phenotypes. Understanding these correlations can help in anticipating disease progression and planning appropriate interventions.

Examples of Genotype–Phenotype Correlations

- *PD*: Mutations in the *LRRK2* gene are associated with late-onset PD and typically show levodopa-responsive parkinsonism.[14] Genotype–phenotype correlation indicates a higher prevalence of nonmotor symptoms such as autonomic dysfunction and psychiatric symptoms **(Table 4)**. *PINK1* and *PRKN* mutations are linked to early-onset PD with autosomal recessive inheritance.[15] Patients often present with dystonia and hyperreflexia, and the response to dopaminergic therapy is usually excellent.
- *Dystonia*: *TOR1A* (DYT1) mutations are the most common cause of early-onset generalized dystonia **(Table 1)**. Patients typically present with limb-onset dystonia that progresses to generalized dystonia during childhood or adolescence.[16] In *THAP1* (DYT6) mutation, dystonia involves the cervical, laryngeal, and cranial muscles. The onset is usually in adolescence or early adulthood, and the progression can be variable.[17]
- *Chorea*: The CAG repeat expansion in the *HTT* gene causes Huntington's disease (HD), characterized by adult-onset chorea, psychiatric symptoms, and cognitive decline **(Table 3)**. The length of the CAG repeat correlates with the age of onset and severity of the disease.[18] *ADCY5* mutation is associated with early-onset chorea and dystonia, often presenting in infancy with paroxysmal exacerbations. The phenotype includes facial myokymia and episodic dystonia.[19]
- *Ataxia*: Spinocerebellar ataxia type 1 (SCA1) caused by ATXN1 mutations presents with progressive cerebellar ataxia, dysarthria, and oculomotor abnormalities[20] **(Table 2)**. The phenotype may also include peripheral neuropathy and pyramidal signs. Mutations in the *FXN* gene lead to Friedreich's ataxia, characterized by progressive gait and limb ataxia, dysarthria, and often cardiomyopathy and diabetes.[21]

Impact of Genotype–Phenotype Correlation on Diagnostic Testing

Genotype–phenotype correlation facilitates the selection of appropriate diagnostic tests, improving diagnostic accuracy and efficiency.

Gene Panels

Panels targeting specific genes associated with the observed phenotype can be utilized for comprehensive testing. For instance, a patient with early-onset parkinsonism may undergo testing for a panel of genes including *PINK1*, *PRKN*, and *DJ-1*, and several others.[22]

Targeted Sequencing

In cases with a strong clinical suspicion of a particular disorder, targeted sequencing of the implicated gene can provide a rapid and definitive diagnosis.

PHENOTYPIC HETEROGENEITY IN GENETIC DISORDERS

Phenotypic heterogeneity refers to the variability in clinical presentations observed in patients with the same genetic disorder. This phenomenon is particularly notable in MDs, where the same genetic mutation can lead to a wide range of symptoms, severity, and disease course. Phenotypic heterogeneity can complicate diagnosis and treatment but also provides valuable insights into disease mechanisms and potential therapeutic targets.

- *Genetic variability and expressivity*: Genetic mutations often exhibit variable expressivity, meaning the same mutation can result in different clinical features among different individuals. For example, mutations in the *GBA* gene, which are associated with Gaucher disease, can also increase the risk of developing PD.[6]
- *Environmental and epigenetic factors*: Environmental factors, lifestyle, and epigenetic modifications can influence the expression of genetic disorders. For instance, the onset and progression of HD, caused by CAG repeat expansions in the *HTT* gene, can be affected by environmental factors and lifestyle choices, such as physical activity and diet.[23]
- *Modifier genes*: The presence of other genetic variants, known as modifier genes, can alter the clinical presentation of a primary genetic disorder. In MDs like dystonia, mutations in primary genes such as *TOR1A* can be modulated by variations in other genes, leading to differences in severity and symptoms among patients.[24]
- *Age of onset*: The age at which symptoms first appear can vary widely even within the same genetic disorder. For example, early-onset forms of parkinsonism are often associated with mutations in genes like *PRKN*, while late-onset forms might be linked to different genetic factors such as *LRRK2*.[25]
- *Clinical presentation*: The same genetic mutation can lead to different MDs. For instance, mutations in the *ATP1A3* gene can cause a spectrum of disorders including rapid-onset dystonia-parkinsonism, alternating hemiplegia of childhood, and cerebellar ataxia.[26]
- *Overlap with other disorders*: Some genetic mutations associated with MDs can present with overlapping features of other neurological conditions. For example, mutations in the *ATP13A2* gene can lead to Kufor-Rakeb syndrome,[27] which presents with parkinsonism, dementia, and pyramidal signs, blurring the lines between distinct clinical entities.

GENETICS IN TREATMENT OF MOVEMENT DISORDERS

Some genetic MDs are considered to be "treatable" or eminently reversible **(Table 5)**.[28] However, apart from these, genetics offers potential for treatment in several other disorders **(Fig. 3)** as well.

Gene Therapy

- *Direct gene replacement*: Gene therapy approaches aim to replace defective genes with functional copies. For example, clinical trials are underway for delivering functional copies of the *GBA* gene in PD patients.
- *Gene silencing*: Techniques such as ribonucleic acid interference (RNAi) and antisense oligonucleotides (ASOs) are being developed to silence harmful gene mutations. An example is the use of ASOs in HD to reduce the production of mutant huntingtin protein.[29]

TABLE 5: Treatable genetic movement disorders.

Disorder	Gene(s) involved	Inheritance pattern	Key features	Treatment options
Wilson's disease	*ATP7B*	Autosomal recessive	Hepatic dysfunction, neurological symptoms (tremor, dystonia, parkinsonism), Kayser–Fleischer rings	Copper chelation therapy (penicillamine, trientine), zinc
Dopa-responsive dystonia (DRD)	*GCH1, TH, SPR, PTS*	Autosomal dominant	Childhood-onset dystonia, diurnal variation, responsiveness to levodopa	Levodopa
Pantothenate kinase-associated neurodegeneration (PKAN)	*PANK2*	Autosomal recessive	Dystonia, parkinsonism, retinal degeneration, iron accumulation in basal ganglia	Symptomatic treatment, iron chelation (deferiprone)
Menkes disease	*ATP7A*	X-linked recessive	Severe neurodegeneration, connective tissue abnormalities, kinky hair	Copper histidine or copper chloride injections
Hereditary hemochromatosis	*HFE, HJV, TFR2, SLC40A1*	Autosomal recessive	Hyperpigmentation, hepatomegaly, diabetes mellitus, cardiomyopathy, arthritis	Phlebotomy, iron chelation therapy
Gaucher disease	*GBA*	Autosomal recessive	Hepatosplenomegaly, bone pain and fractures, anemia, thrombocytopenia, neurological symptoms in type 2 and 3	Enzyme replacement therapy (imiglucerase), substrate reduction therapy (miglustat)
Fabry disease	*GLA*	X-linked recessive	Pain crises, angiokeratomas, corneal opacities, renal failure, cardiomyopathy	Enzyme replacement therapy (agalsidase alpha/beta), chaperone therapy (migalastat)
Biotinidase deficiency	*BTD*	Autosomal recessive	Seizures, hypotonia, ataxia, vision problems, hearing loss, skin rash	Biotin supplementation
Homocystinuria	*CBS, MTHFR, MTR, MTRR, MMADHC*	Autosomal recessive	Marfanoid habitus, lens dislocation, thromboembolism, developmental delay	Vitamin B6, betaine, folic acid, vitamin B12, low-methionine diet, cysteine supplementation
Lesch–Nyhan syndrome	*HPRT1*	X-linked recessive	Self-mutilating behavior, hyperuricemia, gout, renal stones, neurological dysfunction	Allopurinol, febuxostat, symptomatic treatment

Continued

Continued

Disorder	Gene(s) involved	Inheritance pattern	Key features	Treatment options
Niemann–Pick disease	*SMPD1, NPC1, NPC2*	Autosomal recessive	Hepatosplenomegaly, neurological degeneration, lipid storage in cells	Enzyme replacement therapy (olipudase alpha for type B), substrate reduction therapy (miglustat for type C)
Maple syrup urine disease	*BCKDHA, BCKDHB, DBT*	Autosomal recessive	Feeding difficulties, lethargy, developmental delay, sweet-smelling urine	Dietary management, thiamine supplementation
Cystic fibrosis	*CFTR*	Autosomal recessive	Chronic respiratory infections, pancreatic insufficiency, male infertility	CFTR modulators (ivacaftor, lumacaftor, tezacaftor, elexacaftor), symptomatic treatment
Phenylketonuria (PKU)	*PAH*	Autosomal Recessive	Intellectual disability, eczema, seizures, musty odor	Low-phenylalanine diet, sapropterin
Congenital hypothyroidism	*TSHR, DUOX2, DUOXA2, PAX8*	Autosomal recessive	Growth retardation, intellectual disability, jaundice, macroglossia	Thyroid hormone replacement

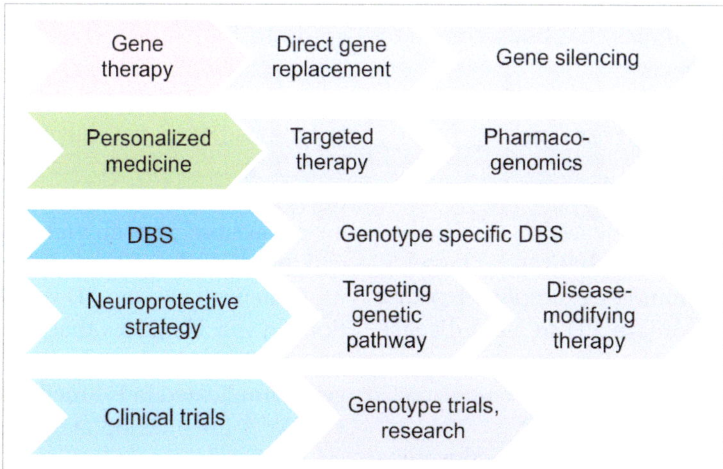

FIG. 3: Genetics in the treatment of movement disorders.

(DBS: deep brain stimulation)

Personalized Medicine

- *Targeted therapies*: Genetic insights have led to the development of targeted therapies that address specific molecular defects. For instance, enzyme replacement therapy for patients with *GBA* mutations in PD.[30]
- *Pharmacogenomics*: Understanding how genetic variations affect drug response has enabled the tailoring of medications to individual genetic profiles, improving efficacy and reducing adverse effects.

Deep Brain Stimulation

Genotype-specific Deep Brain Stimulation

The success of deep brain stimulation (DBS) in treating MDs such as PD and dystonia has been enhanced by understanding the genetic basis of these disorders. Patients with certain genetic profiles, such as those with *LRRK2* mutations, may respond better to DBS, allowing for more personalized treatment strategies. The term "surgicogenomics" has been coined to denote these aspects.[31]

Neuroprotective Strategies

Targeting Genetic Pathways

Research into the genetic causes of MDs has identified key pathways that can be targeted for neuroprotection. For example, targeting the LRRK2 pathway in PD to slow disease progression.[32]

Disease-modifying Therapies

Genetic research has spurred the development of disease-modifying therapies that go beyond symptom management to alter the course of the disease. This includes drugs that target the underlying genetic mutations or their downstream effects.

Clinical Trials and Research

Genotype-based Clinical Trials

The stratification of patients based on genetic profiles has improved the design and outcomes of clinical trials. This approach ensures that therapies are tested on the most relevant patient populations, increasing the likelihood of success.

Collaborative Research Initiatives

Large-scale collaborative initiatives, such as the International Parkinson and Movement Disorder Society Genetics Task Force,[33] have facilitated the sharing of genetic data and resources, accelerating the pace of discovery and translation into clinical practice.

DEEP BRAIN STIMULATION IN GENETICALLY DRIVEN PARKINSON'S DISEASE

Deep brain stimulation has emerged as a highly effective therapeutic intervention for PD, including cases with a genetic basis. While the general principles of DBS apply to both idiopathic and genetic PD, understanding the specific genetic mutations can influence the approach to DBS and its outcomes. Here, we delve into the role of DBS in genetically driven PD, focusing on the relevant genetic mutations, their impact on disease progression and response to DBS, and the clinical implications.

Genetically driven PD is caused by mutations in specific genes that affect the normal functioning of the brain's motor circuitry. Key genes implicated in PD include:[34]

- *SNCA*: Encodes alpha-synuclein, a protein that aggregates in Lewy bodies.
- *LRRK2*: Encodes leucine-rich repeat kinase 2, involved in neuronal signaling.
- *PRKN (parkin)*: Encodes an E3 ubiquitin-protein ligase, involved in protein degradation.

- *PINK1*: Encodes PTEN-induced kinase 1, involved in mitochondrial function.
- *DJ-1*: Encodes a protein involved in oxidative stress response.
- *GBA*: Encodes glucocerebrosidase, involved in lysosomal function and associated with Gaucher disease.

Impact of Genetic Mutations on Deep Brain Stimulation Outcomes

- *SNCA mutation*: Patients with *SNCA* mutations often exhibit early-onset PD with prominent nonmotor symptoms such as cognitive impairment and autonomic dysfunction. While motor symptoms can respond well to DBS, the presence of severe nonmotor symptoms may limit the overall benefits.[35] These patients may experience less improvement in quality of life compared to those with idiopathic PD.
- *LRRK2 mutation*: *LRRK2*-related PD typically presents with a late-onset, slow progression, and often resembles idiopathic PD. Patients with *LRRK2* mutations generally respond well to DBS, with significant improvement in motor symptoms.[36] The response is comparable to that seen in idiopathic PD, making DBS a viable option for these patients.
- *PRKN mutation*: *PRKN* mutations are associated with early-onset PD, often before the age of 40 years, and are characterized by dystonia and hyperreflexia. DBS in *PRKN*-related PD is highly effective, especially in reducing motor fluctuations and dyskinesias. The early-onset and relatively pure motor phenotype make these patients excellent candidates for DBS.[37]
- *PINK1 and DJ-1 mutation*: Both *PINK1* and *DJ-1* mutations result in early-onset PD with a slow progression. Patients often exhibit a good response to levodopa. Similar to *PRKN*-related PD, patients with *PINK1* and *DJ-1* mutations generally show a favorable response to DBS, particularly in terms of motor symptom relief.[38]
- *GBA mutation*: *GBA* mutations are associated with a higher risk of cognitive decline and psychiatric symptoms in addition to the typical motor symptoms of PD. While motor symptoms improve with DBS, the presence of cognitive and psychiatric issues can affect the overall benefit.[39] Careful patient selection and management of nonmotor symptoms are crucial for optimizing outcomes.

Clinical Implications

- *Patient selection*: Genetic testing can help identify patients with specific mutations who are likely to benefit from DBS. It also aids in counseling patients about the expected outcomes and potential challenges. Patients with predominantly motor symptoms and fewer nonmotor symptoms are ideal candidates for DBS. Those with significant cognitive impairment or psychiatric symptoms may require a more nuanced approach.
- *Surgical site considerations*: The choice of target [subthalamic nucleus (STN) vs. globus pallidus internus (GPi)] may vary based on the patient's symptom profile and genetic background. For instance, STN-DBS is often preferred for its effectiveness in reducing motor symptoms and medication dosage, while GPi-DBS may be considered in cases with prominent dystonia.[40]
- *Postoperative management*: Post-DBS, patients often require adjustments in their medication regimen. This is particularly relevant for genetically driven PD, where the response to medications can vary. Continuous monitoring and management of nonmotor symptoms, such as cognitive decline and psychiatric issues, are crucial for maximizing the benefits of DBS.

- *Long-term outcomes*: Understanding the genetic basis of PD can provide insights into the long-term outcomes of DBS. For example, patients with *LRRK2* mutations may experience a more sustained benefit from DBS compared to those with *SNCA* mutations.

DEEP BRAIN STIMULATION IN GENETICALLY-DRIVEN DYSTONIA

The response to pallidal DBS has been observed to vary with the type of monogenic dystonia. DYT-TOR1A (DYT1), which is the most frequent form of monogenic dystonia, has very good outcomes following DBS. The response may be sustained for up to 10 years.[41]

The benefit may be limited in patients who have longer duration of disease and fixed deformities. Secondary worsening has been reported in a subgroup with younger onset and rapid progression.[42]

Good outcomes have also been reported for myoclonus-dystonia syndrome, DYT-*SGCE* (DYT11), and X-linked dystonia-parkinsonism (DYT3). DYT11 is an autosomal dominant condition, with childhood-onset action myoclonus combined with dystonia. Both myoclonus and dystonia improve with DBS, although associated psychiatric comorbidities may not benefit. GPi and ventral intermediate nucleus (VIM) thalamus have been used as DBS targets, with the former being preferred. DYT3 or Lubag (DYT/PARK-TAF1) affects individuals from the Panay island of Philippines.[43] Dystonia tends to be very severe. Both dystonia and parkinsonism improve with DBS.

In contrast, DYT-THAP1 (DYT6) may have more variable outcomes, with improvement, delayed worsening, and nonresponse reported.[44] Variable results have also been reported for other monogenic forms, in smaller case series, including DYT-*KMT2B* (DYT28), DYT-*GNAL* (DYT25), and DYT-*ANO3* (DYT24). Atypical pantothenate kinase-associated neurodegeneration (PKAN) may also respond to pallidal DBS to some extent. These observations are summarized in **Table 6**.

LIMITATIONS OF GENETIC TESTING IN MOVEMENT DISORDERS

The yield of genetic testing in complex MD cohorts has been determined to vary from 21 to 32%, with higher yield for ataxia, moderate for dystonia, and lowest for PD. Due to their broader coverage, WGS and WES have better yield than targeted gene panel testing. WGS may be able to cover intronic regions,

TABLE 6: Response to deep brain stimulation (DBS) in monogenic dystonias.

Gene	Phenotype	DBS response
TOR1A (DYT1)	Early-onset generalized dystonia	Robust response to GPi-DBS, significant reduction in dystonic movements
THAP1 (DYT6)	Mixed dystonia, cranio-cervical involvement, speech difficulties	Substantial improvements, variable response; GPi-DBS effective
GNAL (DYT25)	Adult-onset cervical dystonia, oromandibular dystonia	Good response to GPi-DBS, notable improvement in neck postures and pain
TUBB4A (DYT4)	Whispering dysphonia, generalized dystonia	Positive outcomes with DBS, particularly in reducing generalized symptoms

Continued

Continued

Gene	Phenotype	DBS response
KMT2B (DYT28)	Childhood-onset generalized dystonia, developmental delay	Significant motor improvement with early intervention via DBS
ANO3 (DYT24)	Cranio-cervical or laryngeal dystonia	Substantial benefits from GPi-DBS, improved speech function
GCH1 (DYT5a)	Dopa-responsive dystonia, lower limb involvement	Primary treatment with levodopa; DBS considered if medication response is inadequate
ATP1A3 (DYT12)	Rapid-onset dystonia-parkinsonism	Good response to DBS, significant symptom alleviation
PNKD (DYT8)	Paroxysmal nonkinesigenic dyskinesia, episodic dystonia	Possible reductions in episode frequency and severity with DBS
SLC2A1 (DYT18)	Paroxysmal exercise-induced dyskinesia, GLUT1 deficiency	Some response to DBS, glucose supplementation remains primary treatment

(GPi: globus pallidus internus)

and detect structural variations and repeat expansion disorders better than WES.

However, there are many limitations associated with NGS, including characterization of GC-rich regions, complex structural variants, etc., some of which may be overcome by the use of the upcoming long-read sequencing. Another challenge is when NGS results reveal a variant of uncertain significance (VUS) which are variants that cannot be classified as either pathogenic/likely pathogenic or benign/likely benign. This results in uncertainty among patients and clinicians. Reclassification may be achieved by using in-silico prediction analyses or the use of familial segregation. However, functional studies may be required which are not widely available. Although increasingly affordable, genetic testing continues to be expensive in several parts of the world.

CONCLUSION

The role of genetics seems to be expanding in etiological and therapeutic considerations of MDs. The advent of NGS has permitted analysis of massive amounts of genetic data in parallel, uncovering new genetic discoveries and novel genotype-phenotype correlations. The field of surgicogenomics is advancing, with genetic etiology being used as a predictor of surgical response to DBS. The identification of new genes provides insights into the biological pathways involved in MDs, revealing potential targets for therapeutic intervention. However, it is also increasingly recognized that genetics along may not be sufficient to explain clinical heterogeneity often seen in practice, and there is a definite role for epigenetic factors interacting with the genetic mutation to eventually produce the final clinical picture.

REFERENCES

1. Seaby EG, Pengelly RJ, Ennis S. Exome sequencing explained: a practical guide to its clinical application. Brief Funct Genomics. 2016;15(5): 374-84.
2. Brlek P, Bulić L, Bračić M, Projić P, Škaro V, Shah N, et al. Implementing Whole Genome Sequencing (WGS) in Clinical Practice: Advantages, Challenges, and Future Perspectives. Cells. 2024;13(6):504.
3. Pei XM, Yeung MHY, Wong ANN, Tsang HF, Yu ACS, Yim AKY, et al. Targeted Sequencing approach and its clinical applications for the molecular diagnosis of human diseases. Cells. 2023;12(3):493.

4. Nuytemans K, Theuns J, Cruts M, Van Broeckhoven C. Genetic etiology of Parkinson disease associated with mutations in the SNCA, PARK2, PINK1, PARK7, and LRRK2 genes: a mutation update. Hum Mutat. 2010;31(7):763-80.
5. Zech M, Winkelmann J. Next-generation sequencing and bioinformatics in rare movement disorders. Nat Rev Neurol. 2024;20:114-26.
6. Riboldi GM, Di Fonzo AB. GBA, Gaucher Disease, and Parkinson's Disease: From Genetic to Clinic to New Therapeutic Approaches. Cells. 2019;8(4):364.
7. Singh B, Xu J, Wang H. VPS13C deficiency in the context of Parkinson's disease: linking lysosomal dysfunction to neurodegeneration. Acta Neuropathol Commun. 2021;9(1):133.
8. Carecchio M, Mencacci NE, Iodice A, Pons R, Panteghini C, Zorzi G, et al. ADCY5-related movement disorders: Frequency, disease course and phenotypic variability in a cohort of paediatric patients. Parkinsonism Relat Disord. 2017;41:37-43.
9. Ciarleglio LJ, Bennett RL, Williamson J, Mandell JB, Marks JH. Genetic counseling throughout the life cycle. J Clin Invest. 2003;112(9):1280-6.
10. Koptielow J, Szyłak E, Szewczyk-Roszczenko O, Roszczenko P, Kochanowicz J, Kułakowska A, et al. Genetic Update and Treatment for Dystonia. Int J Mol Sci. 2024;25(7):3571.
11. Sandford E, Burmeister M. Genes and genetic testing in hereditary ataxias. Genes (Basel). 2014;5(3):586-603.
12. Mencacci NE, Carecchio M. Recent advances in genetics of chorea. Curr Opin Neurol. 2016;29(4):486-95.
13. Day JO, Mullin S. The Genetics of Parkinson's Disease and Implications for Clinical Practice. Genes. 2021;12(7):1006.
14. Wider C, Dickson DW, Wszolek ZK. Leucine-rich repeat kinase 2 gene-associated disease: redefining genotype-phenotype correlation. Neurodegener Dis. 2010;7(1-3):175-9.
15. Brooks J, Ding J, Simon-Sanchez J, Paisan-Ruiz C, Singleton AB, Scholz SW. Parkin and PINK1 mutations in early-onset Parkinson's disease: comprehensive screening in publicly available cases and control. J Med Genet. 2009;46(6):375-81.
16. Koptielow J, Szyłak E, Szewczyk-Roszczenko O, Roszczenko P, Kochanowicz J, Kułakowska A, et al. Genetic Update and Treatment for Dystonia. Int J Mol Sci. 2024;25(7):3571.
17. LeDoux MS, Xiao J, Rudzińska M, Bastian RW, Wszolek ZK, Van Gerpen JA, et al. Genotype-phenotype correlations in THAP1 dystonia: molecular foundations and description of new cases. Parkinsonism Relat Disord. 2012;18(5):414-25.
18. Jiang A, Handley RR, Lehnert K, Snell RG. From Pathogenesis to Therapeutics: A Review of 150 Years of Huntington's Disease Research. Int J Mol Sci. 2023;24(16):13021.
19. Chang FCF, Westenberger A, Dale RC, Smith M, Pall HS, Perez-Dueñas B, et al. Phenotypic insights into ADCY5-associated disease. Mov Disord. 2016;31:1033-40.
20. Suart CE, Perez AM, Al-Ramahi I, Maiuri T, Botas J, Truant R. Spinocerebellar Ataxia Type 1 protein Ataxin-1 is signaled to DNA damage by ataxia-telangiectasia mutated kinase. Hum Mol Genet. 2021;30(8):706-15.
21. Cook A, Giunti P. Friedreich's ataxia: clinical features, pathogenesis and management. Br Med Bull. 2017;124(1):19-30.
22. Klein C. Implications of genetics on the diagnosis and care of patients with parkinson disease. Arch Neurol. 2006;63(3):328-34.
23. Calluori S, Stark R, Pearson BL. Gene-Environment Interactions in Repeat Expansion Diseases: Mechanisms of Environmentally Induced Repeat Instability. Biomedicines. 2023;11(2):515.
24. Saffari A, Lau T, Tajsharghi H, Karimiani EG, Kariminejad A, Efthymiou S, et al. The clinical and genetic spectrum of autosomal-recessive TOR1A-related disorders. Brain. 2023;146(8):3273-88.
25. Correia Guedes L, Mestre T, Outeiro TF, Ferreira JJ. Are genetic and idiopathic forms of Parkinson's disease the same disease? J Neurochem. 2020;152(5):515-22.
26. Vezyroglou A, Akilapa R, Barwick K, Koene S, Brownstein CA, Holder-Espinasse M, et al. The Phenotypic Continuum of ATP1A3-Related Disorders. Neurology. 2022;99(14):e1511-26.
27. Kola S, Meka SSL, Syed TF, Kandadai RM, Alugolu R, Borgohain R. Kufor–Rakeb Syndrome with Novel Mutation and the Role of Deep Brain Stimulation. Mov Disord Clin Pract. 2022;9(6):1003-7.
28. Jinnah HA, Albanese A, Bhatia KP, Cardoso F, Da Prat G, de Koning TJ, et al. Treatable inherited rare movement disorders. Mov Disord. 2018;33(1):21-35.
29. Wild EJ, Tabrizi SJ. Therapies targeting DNA and RNA in Huntington's disease. Lancet Neurol. 2017;16(10):837-47.

30. Chen Y, Sam R, Sharma P, Chen L, Do J, Sidransky E. Glucocerebrosidase as a therapeutic target for Parkinson's disease. Expert Opin Ther Targets. 2020;24(4):287-94.
31. Visanji NP, Ghani M, Yu E, Kakhki EG, Sato C, Moreno D, et al. Axial Impairment Following Deep Brain Stimulation in Parkinson's Disease: A Surgicogenomic Approach. J Parkinsons Dis. 2022;12(1):117-28.
32. Taymans JM, Fell M, Greenamyre T, Hirst WD, Mamais A, Padmanabhan S, et al. Perspective on the current state of the LRRK2 field. NPJ Parkinsons Dis. 2023;9:104.
33. Lange LM, Gonzalez-Latapi P, Rajalingam R, Tijssen MAJ, Ebrahimi-Fakhari D, Gabbert C, et al. Nomenclature of Genetic Movement Disorders: Recommendations of the International Parkinson and Movement Disorder Society Task Force–An Update. Mov Disord. 2022;37(5):905-35.
34. França C, Carra RB, Diniz JM, Munhoz RP, Cury RG. Deep brain stimulation in Parkinson's disease: state of the art and future perspectives. Arq Neuropsiquiatr. 2022;80(5 Suppl 1):105-15.
35. Fouarge E, Garraux G, Kaschten B, Salado AL, Parmentier E. One-Year Follow-Up of Subthalamic Nucleus Deep Brain Stimulation in SNCA Mutation Parkinsonism: A Case Report. Tremor Other Hyperkinet Mov (N Y). 2023;13:47.
36. Chen S, Liu H, Wu QQ, Xu SJ, Li WG, Chen T, et al. Effect of LRRK2 G2385R Variant on Subthalamic Deep Brain Stimulation Efficacy in Parkinson's Disease in a Han Chinese Population. Front Neurol. 2019;10:1231.
37. Zhu W, Huang X, Yoon E, Bandres-Ciga S, Blauwendraat C, Billingsley KJ, et al. Heterozygous PRKN mutations are common but do not increase the risk of Parkinson's disease. Brain. 2022;145(6):2077-91.
38. Cookson MR. Parkinsonism due to mutations in PINK1, parkin, and DJ-1 and oxidative stress and mitochondrial pathways. Cold Spring Harb Perspect Med. 2012;2(9):a009415.
39. Clark LN, Ross BM, Wang Y, Mejia-Santana H, Harris J, Louis ED, et al. Mutations in the glucocerebrosidase gene are associated with early-onset Parkinson disease. Neurology. 2007;69:1270-7.
40. Williams NR, Foote KD, Okun MS. STN vs. GPi Deep Brain Stimulation: Translating the Rematch into Clinical Practice. Mov Disord Clin Pract. 2014;1(1):24-35.
41. Tisch S, Kumar KR. Pallidal Deep Brain Stimulation for Monogenic Dystonia: The Effect of Gene on Outcome. Front Neurol. 2021;11:630391.
42. Hale AT, Monsour MA, Rolston JD, Naftel RP, Englot DJ. Deep brain stimulation in pediatric dystonia: a systematic review. Neurosurg Rev. 2020;43(3):873-80.
43. Lee LV, Munoz EL, Tan KT, Reyes MT. Sex linked recessive dystonia parkinsonism of Panay, Philippines (XDP). Mol Pathol. 2001;54(6):362-8.
44. Danielsson A, Carecchio M, Cif L, Koy A, Lin JP, Solders G, et al. Pallidal Deep Brain Stimulation in DYT6 Dystonia: Clinical Outcome and Predictive Factors for Motor Improvement. J Clin Med. 2019;8(12):2163.

CHAPTER 11

Diagnosis and Management of Autoimmune Movement Disorders

Sayooja Sachithanandan, Asish Vijayaraghavan, Divya Kalikavil Puthanveedu, Syam Krishnan

ABSTRACT

Neuroimmunology is a rapidly evolving field. The discovery of newer antibodies and syndromes continuously expands the clinical spectrum and our understanding of the pathophysiology and treatment of autoimmune neurological disorders. Movement disorders are common in autoantibody-associated neurological diseases. This is a category of potentially treatable conditions, and differentiation from metabolic, infectious, or neurodegenerative disorders, which they mimic, is vital for this reason. Acquired movement disorders resulting from immune-mediated mechanisms require early recognition due to their treatment implications. The autoantibodies behave differently in their response to therapy and association with malignancy, based on their antigenic targets being extracellular, synaptic intracellular, or cytoplasmic. Awareness regarding distinct clinical features characteristic of specific autoimmune movement disorders (AMDs) is essential for clinicians to enable precise antibody testing and prompt treatment initiation. This review classifies AMDs as primary and secondary and describes the antibodies associated with primary AMDs. The salient features of major AMDs, phenomenology-based approach, and decision-making protocols based on the presence and type of autoantibodies are elaborated further, thereby providing a practical guide for evaluating and managing AMDs.

Keywords: Movement disorders, Autoimmune, Paraneoplastic, Autoantibodies.

INTRODUCTION

Autoimmune movement disorders (AMDs) are an evolving and heterogeneous group of conditions, with an increasing number of syndromes and autoantibodies being discovered. Movement disorders are probably the most noticeable symptoms in neuroimmunology, bringing the patient to the physician. Autoimmune causes are reported in up to 42% of children with acute movement disorders.[1] AMDs often coexist with limbic encephalitis, epilepsy, or peripheral neuropathy. Early diagnosis is crucial because some antibodies are associated with occult neoplasia, which can be potentially treatable. However, many patients are diagnosed late or often misdiagnosed. Although certain movement disorders can form classic syndromes pointing toward specific autoantibodies, clinical diagnosis is often challenging because of the overlapping presentations and often undetectable antibodies.

CLASSIFICATION OF AUTOIMMUNE MOVEMENT DISORDERS

Clinical conditions manifesting as movement disorders (hypo- or hyperkinetic) and resulting from an autoimmune etiology are termed AMDs.[2] They can be arbitrarily classified into two groups:

1. *Primary AMDs:* These are caused by autoantibodies, usually triggered by infections or neoplasms and primarily targeting the central nervous system (CNS), including the nodes of the neural circuits concerned with motor control. The antigenic targets could be extracellular, synaptic intracellular, or cytoplasmic. This group includes various autoimmune encephalitis (AIE) syndromes and paraneoplastic encephalitis manifesting as movement disorders.[3,4]
2. *Secondary AMD:* This group is constituted by systemic autoimmune conditions causing movement disorders secondary to nervous system affliction. These are usually associated with prominent extraneurological manifestations. Immune-mediated primary CNS demyelinating disorders like multiple sclerosis (MS) sometimes cause movement disorders secondary to damage to basal ganglia or cerebellar circuits and these also could be considered as secondary AMDs.[5]

CLASSIFICATION OF AUTOANTIBODIES

As discussed above, the autoantibodies causing AMDs can be targeted toward extracellular, synaptic intracellular, or cytoplasmic antigens. Characterization of autoantibodies in primary AMDs based on immunological mechanisms targeting different cellular components has treatment implications.[2,6,7] Autoantibodies against the neuronal cell surface receptors cause receptor dysfunction, which is usually reversible, leading to dysregulation of downstream mechanisms and manifesting as hyperkinetic movement disorders, seizures, or cognitive decline. They exert pathogenicity through antibody-mediated mechanisms such as antigen internalization, direct agonist or antagonist effects on receptors and activation of the complement cascade, or through cell-mediated cytotoxicity leading to neuronal damage.[1] These disorders have, in general, a favorable response to immunotherapy and when they occur in a paraneoplastic setting, treatment of the underlying neoplasm.[2,8]

The second group of autoantibodies target antigens localized to the presynaptic intracellular region and interferes with the release of inhibitory neurotransmitters. These commonly manifest as ataxia and Stiff-person phenotype. They have an intermediate response to immunotherapy.[2] The third group is composed of onconeural antibodies targeting the cytoplasmic and nuclear antigens, highly associated with malignancies and presenting as paraneoplastic syndromes of the varied clinical picture. Such antibodies directed against intracellular components are useful as biomarkers of the disease and aid diagnosis but are usually not causative because there is no opportunity for the antibodies to bind to the intracellular targets. The associated diseases are thought to be mediated by autoreactive T cells and this group is poorly responsive to immunotherapy.[8,9] Examples of AMDs under each category of autoantibodies are mentioned in **Table 1**.

TABLE 1: Salient features of antibodies directed against different cell targets.

Autoantibody target	Neuronal cell surface receptors (B cell-mediated)	Intracellular synaptic proteins	Cytoplasmic and nuclear antigens (T cell-mediated)
Usual clinical features	Seizures, cognitive dysfunction, orolingual dyskinesias, ataxia, and parkinsonism	Ataxia, Stiff-person syndrome	Ataxia, limbic encephalitis
Prototype antigen target examples	NMDARE, LGI1, CASPR2, DPPX, Dopamine-2-R, IgLON5, GABAAR, GABABR, VGCC, mGluR1, mGluR5, Neurexin-3α, and AQP4	GAD, amphiphysin, GlyR, Gephyrin, and GABARAP	Hu, CV2/CRMP5, Yo, Ma, Ri, Zic4, PCA2, Sox1, GFAP
Association with malignancy	Low and variable	Moderate	High
Response to immunotherapy	Favorable	Moderate	Poor

(AQP4: aquaporin-4; CASPR2: contactin-associated protein-like 2; CV2/CRMP5: collapsin response-mediator protein 5; DPPX: dipeptidylpeptidase-like protein-6; GABAAR: γ-aminobutyric acid A receptor; GABABR: γ-aminobutyric acid B receptor; GAD: glutamic acid decarboxylase; GFAP: glial fibrillary acidic protein; GlyR: glycine receptor; IgLON5: immunoglobulin-like cell adhesion molecule 5; LGI1: leucine-rich glioma-inactivated 1; mGLuR1: metabotropic glutamate receptor type 1; mGLuR5: metabotropic glutamate receptor type 5; NMDARE: N-methyl-D-aspartate receptor encephalitis; PCA2: Purkinje cell antibody 2; SOX1: Sry-like high mobility group box 1; VGCC: voltage-gated calcium channel; Zic4: zinc finger domain of the intracellular transcription factor)

AUTOIMMUNE MOVEMENT DISORDERS WITH WELL-CHARACTERIZED ANTIBODIES AND CLINICAL PHENOTYPES

The characteristic features of some important AMDs are mentioned below. A description of different autoantibody-mediated syndromes is also summarized in **Table 2.**[10-42]

Anti-N-methyl-D-aspartate Receptor Encephalitis

N-methyl-D-aspartate receptor encephalitis (NMDARE) was identified to be more than four times as frequent as viral encephalitis in the California Encephalitis Project and was considered the single most common cause of encephalitis in individuals under the age of 30 years.[10] NMDARE exhibits a myriad of movement disorders of which orolingual, facial, and lingual dyskinesias are the most characteristic **(Table 2)**. Isolated movement disorder presentation is rare; patients mostly present with subacute onset psychiatric or cognitive dysfunction, speech disturbances including mutism, seizures, autonomic dysfunction, central hypoventilation, hyperkinetic movement disorders, and altered sensorium which form the six major groups of symptoms.[3,8] They often exhibit an age-dependent clinical presentation.[7,11] Children are more likely to develop movement disorders and seizures, which are generally refractory to symptomatic therapy and improve gradually with recovery from the disease following immunotherapy,[1] while adults mostly have neuropsychiatric and behavioral disturbances. Prodromal fever and headache are reported by many patients. The disease is mostly idiopathic; sometimes, it can be triggered by either malignancy (particularly, ovarian teratoma in young women) or infection like herpes simplex encephalitis.[12] The diagnostic criteria offer two levels of certainty. Definite NMDARE requires the presence of cerebrospinal fluid (CSF) antibodies against the glycine

TABLE 2: Autoantibodies, associated autoimmune movement disorders (AMDs), and other clinical features.

Antigen target	Demographics	Movement disorders	Other clinical features	Tumor association	Ancillary investigations
NMDARE[1,2,8,30]	Young women (15–40 years) and children	Orofacial and lingual dyskinesias, dystonia, stereotypies, chorea, myorhythmia, and cerebellar ataxia	Altered sensorium, seizures, catatonia, speech dysfunction, memory decline, central hypoventilation, and dysautonomia	Ovarian teratoma, lung, and testicular carcinoma	Extreme delta brush in EEG. T2/FLAIR signal hyperintensities in the hippocampus, temporal cortex, frontal cortex, and brainstem. Anti-NMDARE antibodies demonstrated in CSF have higher sensitivity than in serum
LGI-1[1,2,31]	More common in males; typical age—sixth and seventh decades	FBDS, chorea, myoclonus, dystonia, and parkinsonism	Amnesia, seizures, personality changes, psychosis, sleep disorders, Morvan syndrome, and neuropathic pain	Thymoma	Hyponatremia in 70% of patients. Episodic bradycardia in ECG. Serological studies are more sensitive than CSF for *LGI1* antibodies. Hyperintensities in T2-weighted MR images in the mesial temporal lobe
CAPSR2[1,2,30,37]	Much more common in males (sex ratio 8:1). Typical age—fifth and sixth decades	Ataxia, chorea, orthostatic myoclonus, trunk flexion myoclonus superficially resembling psychogenic propriospinal myoclonus, parkinsonism	Morvan syndrome, neuropathic pain, limbic encephalitis, and seizures	Thymoma, prostate and lung cancer, and melanoma	Nonspecific inflammatory changes in CSF and MRI. Neuromyotonia, fasciculations, and myokymic discharges in EMG. Serum assessments are highly sensitive for *CASPR2* antibodies
DPPX[1,37]	More common in males in fifth and sixth decades	Hyperekplexia, tremor, myoclonus, SPS, PERM, ataxia, and PLMS	Prolonged diarrhea, weight loss, seizures, psychiatric symptoms, dysautonomia, and intractable pruritus	B-cell lymphoma	Normal MRI. Anti-DPPX detectable in both serum and CSF

Continued

Continued

Antigen target	Demographics	Movement disorders	Other clinical features	Tumor association	Ancillary investigations
GABAAR[1,30,38]	Young males, median age of 41 years, range from 17 to 73 years	Dystonic tongue movements, chorea, opsoclonus, ataxia, and orofacial dyskinesias	Seizures (most prominent), status epilepticus, and encephalopathy	Hodgkin's lymphoma	MRI—Multifocal T2-FLAIR cortical-subcortical hyperintensities involving cingulate, temporal (95%), and frontal (65%) regions, basal ganglia, cerebellum, and brainstem
GABABR[1,39]	Equal gender distribution, Usual age: 40–50 years	Ataxia, chorea, and opsoclonus	Refractory status epilepticus, encephalopathy,and limbic encephalitis syndrome	SCLC	• Brainstem, basal ganglia, and mesial temporal lobe hyperintensities in MRI • Concurrent GAD antibody positivity can occur
D2R[1,40]	Equal gender distribution. Usually affects children; Median age: 10 years	Basal ganglia encephalitis manifesting as generalized or hemidystonia, parkinsonism, oculogyric crisis, chorea and tics	Psychiatric symptoms, seizures, ocular flutter, and encephalopathy	None	T2-FLAIR hyperintensities within the basal ganglia, in MRI
KLH11[37]	Usually affect males. Age range: 9–72 years	Ataxia and OMAS	Hearing loss, cognitive decline, limbic encephalitis syndrome, and psychosis	Testicular seminoma, ovarian teratoma	Nonspecific inflammatory changes in CSF and MRI
GAD[2]	Middle-aged females	Ataxia, palatal myoclonus, and PERM	SPS, episodic vertigo, limbic encephalitis, seizures. Can be comorbid with type 1 diabetes and thyroiditis	SCLC and thymoma	CSF anti-GAD antibodies are usually positive. EMG shows continuous agonist and antagonist motor activity, typically in axial muscles. Epileptiform discharges in EEG. Normal or showing bilateral T2-FLAIR mesial temporal hyperintensities in MRI

Continued

Continued

Antigen target	Demographics	Movement disorders	Other clinical features	Tumor association	Ancillary investigations
GlyR[30]	No gender predilection, wide age range of 1–75 years	SPS and PERM	Epilepsy, brainstem, autonomic, and long-tract signs	Thymoma, SCLC, and breast cancer	Nonspecific inflammatory changes in CSF and MRI
Amphiphysin[30]	Females, median age 52 years	SPS and ataxia	Sensory neuronopathy, myelopathy and limbic encephalitis syndrome	Breast and lung cancer	Nonspecific inflammatory changes in CSF and MRI
GFAP astrocytopathy[30,41]	No gender predilection, median age: 42 years	Tremor and ataxia	Meningoencephalitis, myelitis, headache, papilledema and subacute encephalopathy	Prostate and gastrointestinal adenocarcinoma, melanoma, myeloma	Characteristic MRI findings—radial, linear periventricular, or cerebellar gadolinium enhancement
Hu[30]	Middle-aged and older adult males	Chorea, opsoclonus-myoclonus, and pseudoathetosis	Sensory neuronopathy, limbic encephalitis, rhombencephalitis, gastrointestinal pseudo-obstruction, sensorineural hearing loss	Small cell lung cancer	Anti-Hu antibodies in both serum and CSF. Nonspecific inflammatory changes in CSF and MRI. Epileptiform discharges in EEG, FDG-PET shows extensive bilateral mesial temporal hypermetabolism
Ri[30]	More in women aged more than 45 years	Cranio-cervical dystonia (jaw closing or opening dystonia), cerebellar ataxia	Oculomotor disturbances, encephalopathy, and SPS	Breast cancer	Cerebellar atrophy. Nonspecific inflammatory changes in CSF and MRI
CV2/CRMP5[28,30,42]	No gender predilection, 60–70 years	Chorea, dystonia, and ataxia	Limbic encephalitis, optic neuritis, uveitis, myelitis, sensory neuronopathy, anosmia, and ageusia	SCLC, Thymoma, NHL, and breast cancer	Nonspecific inflammatory changes in CSF and MRI
Ma[21,22]	Young males 30–40 years; elderly females aged 60–70 years	Parkinsonism, PSP-like phenotype, cataplexy, and cerebellar ataxia	Weight gain, limbic, diencephalic, and brainstem encephalitis, myelopathy, radiculo-plexopathy, and sleep disorders like RBD	Testicular malignancy, SCLC, and breast cancer	Typical MRI pattern with thalamic and hypothalamic T2 hyperintensities

Continued

Continued

Antigen target	Demographics	Movement disorders	Other clinical features	Tumor association	Ancillary investigations
PDE10A[11,30]	No gender predilection, median age: 70 years	Chorea, dystonia, and ballismus	Encephalopathy	SCLC and renal adenocarcinoma	Nonspecific inflammatory changes in CSF and MRI, bilateral striatal lesions
IgLON5[16-20]	No gender predilection, Age: 40–70 years	Characteristic NREM parasomnia (finalistic movements), RBD, abdominal; dyskinesia, parkinsonism, ataxia, dystonia, chorea, myoclonus, and SPS	Prominent sleep dysfunction, OSA, bulbar dysfunction, motor neuron disease, supranuclear gaze palsy	None	PSG demonstrates OSA, complex non-REM parasomnia, and stridor during sleep. Anti-*IgLON5* detected in serum and CSF (IgG4 or IgG1). CSF antibodies more specific. Associated with human leukocyte markers HLA-DRB1*10:01 and HLADQB1*05:01. Neuropathology demonstrates accumulation of hyperphosphorylated tau, preferentially in the hypothalamus and brainstem tegmental nuclei
SEZ6L2[11]	No gender predilection, median age 62 years	Cerebellar ataxia and atypical parkinsonism	Cognitive impairment, dysarthria	None	Mostly normal CSF and MRI brain. Antibodies of IgG4 class predominantly
mGluR5[11,28]	Females, median age 30 years	Myoclonus, dystonia, orofacial dyskinesias, and postural tremors	Neuropsychiatric symptoms, Ophelia syndrome (encephalitis, memory deficits, and dreamy state)	SCLC and Hodgkin's lymphoma	Nonspecific inflammatory changes in CSF and MRI

(CASPR2: contactin-associated protein-like 2; CSF: cerebrospinal fluid; D2R: dopamine receptor type 2; DPPX: dipeptidylpeptidase-like protein-6; EEG: electroencephalogram; EMG: electromyogram; FBDS: faciobrachial dystonic seizures; FDG-PET: [^{18}F]Fluorodeoxyglucose positron emission tomography; FLAIR: fluid-attenuation inversion recovery; IgLON5: immunoglobulin-like cell adhesion molecule-5; GABAAR: γ-aminobutyric acid A receptor; GAD: glutamic acid decarboxylase; GFAP: glial fibrillary acidic protein; GlyR: glycine receptor; KLHL11: Kelch-like protein 11; LGI1: leucine-rich glioma-inactivated 1; MRI: magnetic resonance imaging; mGLuR5: metabotropic glutamate receptor type-5; NHL: non-Hodgkins lymphoma; NMDARE: N-methyl-D-aspartate receptor encephalitis; NREM: non-rapid eye movement; OMAS: opsoclonus-myoclonus-ataxia syndrome; OSA: obstructive sleep apnea; PDE10A: phosphodiesterase 10A; PERM: progressive encephalomyelitis with rigidity and myoclonus; PLMS: periodic limb movements in sleep; PSG: polysomnogram; PSP: progressive supranuclear palsy; RBD: rapid eye movement sleep behavioral disorder; SEZ6L2: seizure-related-6-homolog like autoimmunity; SCLC: small cell lung cancer; SPS: Stiff-person syndrome) binding (GluN1) subunit of the receptor to be demonstrated along with one or more of the six major groups of symptoms as mentioned earlier in the text.[3] Probable NMDARE is diagnosed when there are at least four out of six major groups of symptoms, with at least one of the supportive laboratory testing [abnormal electroencephalogram (EEG), CSF pleocytosis, or oligoclonal bands] **(Table 2)**.

Hyperkinetic crisis, dysautonomia, and differentiating true seizures from dyskinesias are potential challenges in management. Although uncommon, initial presentation with gyratory seizures could be an early clue pointing toward this disorder.[13] The anti-NMDAR Encephalitis One-Year Functional Status (NEOS) score is a useful tool for predicting the probability of poor functional outcome at 1 year, where one point each is given for ICU admission, delay in treatment for 4 weeks, absence of improvement within 4 weeks of treatment, abnormal magnetic resonance imaging (MRI), and CSF white blood cell count of >20 cells/μL.[14] Prompt administration of immunotherapy and removal of tumors when present are often rewarding. The treatment decisions should be primarily guided by clinical assessment as CSF antibody titers on follow-up do not correlate with the clinical course. A similar picture of prodromal fever and headache followed by neuropsychiatric disturbances, orofacial dyskinesias, seizures, dysautonomia, and altered sensorium can be present in neurexin 3α antibody-associated disorder.[11,15]

Anti-immunoglobulin-like Cell Adhesion Molecule Family Member-5 Disease

The earliest description of the anti-immunoglobulin-like cell adhesion molecule family member-5 (IgLON5) disease in 2014 came from a Sleep laboratory in Spain, following observation of patients having unique nonrapid eye movement (NREM) and rapid eye movement (REM) parasomnia with sleep breathing dysfunction, gait instability, and brainstem symptoms.[16] Features suggestive of both autoimmune mechanisms [such as anti-IgLON5 autoantibodies and a strong association with specific human leukocyte antigen (HLA)], as well as neurodegenerative diseases (hyperphosphorylated tau accumulations and limited response to immunotherapy), were subsequently reported.[17] The exact pathogenesis of this disorder remains unclear, with ongoing debate as to whether the immune abnormality is the cause or a consequence of a primary neurodegenerative process.[18] This disease, which has no specific gender predisposition, is a great mimicker and can present in older adults with clinical syndromes resembling a chronic degenerative disorder. Presentations with clinical features similar to progressive supranuclear palsy, multiple system atrophy, corticobasal syndrome, and motor neuron disease or with progressive dementia have been described; prominent sleep dysfunction out of proportion to that expected in the typical neurodegenerative syndromes could act as a diagnostic clue **(Table 2)**.[19] The sleep symptoms include NREM parasomnias, specifically "finalistic" movements, and REM parasomnias like REM sleep behavioral disorder (RBD). The IgLON5 composite score (ICS) is a severity assessment tool, which includes 17 symptoms distributed in five domains covering most of the clinical manifestations.[20] As antibodies are predominantly of the IgG4 subclass that is unable to activate complement-mediated immune reaction, poor response with intravenously immunoglobulin (IVIG) monotherapy is expected. Although combination therapy with rituximab, plasmapheresis, and IVIG works better if administered in the early phases, the overall prognosis of anti-IgLON5 disease is poor. A high-serum level of neurofilament light chain at diagnosis would predict a worse prognosis with immunotherapy.[17]

Anti-Ma2/Ma1 Encephalitis

Anti-Ma2/Ma1 encephalitis is a diagnosis that needs to be considered in patients with isolated or combined limbic, diencephalic, or brainstem dysfunction. Ma2 and Ma1 antibodies tend to coexist in the same patient with the above-mentioned combination of clinical features, though Ma2 occurs at a higher frequency.[21] The presence of prominent diencephalic involvement (excessive daytime sleepiness, narcolepsy, or cataplexy) and upper brainstem involvement (e.g., atypical parkinsonism) with MRI abnormalities in the region distinguishes it from other paraneoplastic encephalitis syndromes.[21,22] Primary testicular neoplasm is a common association seen in young males, and lung cancer in the elderly.[21] The presence of additional Ma1 antibodies confers a worse prognosis as they have more extensive brainstem and cerebellar involvement and are associated with nontesticular cancers which, in turn, are more difficult to treat than testicular germ cell tumors. Features favoring improvement or stabilization with immunotherapy in a case of Ma2/Ma1 encephalitis include male gender, age <45 years, testicular tumor with complete response to oncological treatment, absence of anti-Ma1 antibodies, and limited CNS involvement.[21]

Anti-Homer-3 Antibody-mediated Disease

Anti-Homer-3 antibody-mediated disease is increasingly recognized as an autoimmune mimic of the cerebellar type of multiple system atrophy (MSA-C), characterized by cerebellar ataxia. Dysautonomia and REM-sleep behavioral disorders (RBD), with additional features like myeloradiculopathy, and encephalopathy may be seen.[23,24] There is no sex predilection, and the common age group affected is 40–50 years. CSF is mostly abnormal with inflammatory changes, but antibody detection can be challenging as currently available detection techniques have low sensitivity.[24] MRI also could be misleading with cerebellar/pontine atrophy and a "hot-cross bun" sign. They are not associated with malignancies and have variable responses to immunotherapy.[23]

Anti-Kelch-like Protein 11 Syndrome

A recent addition to the multitude of autoantibodies causing AMDs is the anti-Kelch-like protein 11 (KLH 11) syndrome.[25] They present as rapidly progressive ataxia, rhombencephalitis, and cochlea-vestibulopathy, discovered in patients with testicular seminoma.[26] They have poor response to immunotherapy owing to the intracellular nature of the target antigen. A clinical scoring validated termed MATCH (male sex:1 point, ataxia/cerebellar signs: 1 point, testicular tumor: 2 points, or other types of tumors: 1 point, hearing impairment: 1 point) helps in identifying conventional antibody-negative patients suspected to be harboring anti-KLH-11.[27]

Other AMDs include poststreptococcal and other postinfectious movement disorders [Sydenham chorea (SC), pediatric autoimmune neuropsychiatric disorder associated with streptococcal infection (PANDAS)], pediatric acute-onset neuropsychiatric symptoms (PANS) and systemic autoimmune conditions associated movement disorders [Sjögren syndrome, celiac disease, systemic lupus erythematosus (SLE) and antiphospholipid antibody (APLA) syndrome].[5,28] SC which is considered a part of rheumatic fever is the prototype example of acute to subacute childhood choreatic disorder, caused due to autoimmunity triggered by group A streptococcal infection.[29] It may be accompanied by neuropsychiatric morbidities and frequent relapses and remissions. No specific causative antibodies responsible for CNS inflammation have been demonstrated so far. Autoimmune basal ganglia encephalitis is at the rarer spectrum of pediatric AMDs, triggered by mycoplasma, Epstein-Barr virus, influenza, and Group A streptococcal infections.[29] It is characterized by parkinsonism, hyperkinetic movement disorders, sleep and neuropsychiatric disturbances, and autonomic dysfunction along with the presence of oligoclonal bands in CSF, without any evidence for an infective agent and responds to immunomodulation with steroids.[8]

Immune checkpoint inhibitors (ICI) are used for the treatment of cancer and act by neutralizing tumor evading T-cell immune responses. Though more often associated with autoimmune myasthenia, polyradiculoneuropathy, myositis, myelitis, and meningitis, widespread use of ICI is also postulated to be a risk factor for the increasing incidence of AMDs like limbic encephalitis and Ma2 encephalitis.[27,30]

WHEN TO SUSPECT AUTOIMMUNE MOVEMENT DISORDER?

The Graus criteria for AIE may be extrapolated to identify clues to suspect AMDs.[3] Subacute onset (<3 months), rapid progression, and presence of mixed movement disorders, accompanied by seizures, cognitive decline, altered sensorium, evidence for inflammation in CSF or MRI and propensity for autoimmunity or history of neoplasm should raise the suspicion of autoimmunity as a cause of the movement disorder.[3,29] Association with features suggestive of limbic encephalitis, subacute cerebellar degeneration, encephalomyelitis, and sensory neuronopathy also point toward autoimmunity, particularly of paraneoplastic etiology.[9]

Phenomenology in AMDs is difficult to classify due to the mixed presentations and coexisting abnormalities due to multifocal or diffuse involvement of neuraxis and peripheral nervous system (higher-level gait disorders, cerebellar ataxia, peripheral movement disorders like the ones resulting from peripheral nerve hyperexcitability and Stiff-person syndrome, and tremor and pseudoathetosis secondary to peripheral nerve involvement, etc.). It is also tricky sometimes to diagnose movement disorders in the background of active psychosis, irritability, and seizures (e.g., differentiating dystonia from focal tonic seizures in NMDARE). However, certain movement disorder phenomenologies should prompt the clinician to evaluate further for autoimmune etiology.[30]

Dystonia

Faciobrachial dystonic seizure in leucine-rich glioma-inactivated-1 (LGI1) related encephalitis is considered an immune-mediated paroxysmal movement disorder, occurring as brief (less than a few seconds) and frequent (100s/day) episodes of abnormal posturing of ipsilateral face and arm, poorly responsive to antiseizure medication and with a typically normal EEG.[1,30] Jaw dystonia and laryngospasm are typically seen in anti-Ri mediated encephalitis.[31] Dystonia of autoimmune etiology differs from isolated and combined genetic dystonic disorders in its anatomical distribution, age of onset, and temporal profile (generally occur acutely or subacutely) and usually is "combined", forming part of an encephalopathic syndrome, rather than occurring as an isolated manifestation.[7,30] AIE should be a differential diagnosis in the evaluation of dystonia with encephalopathy, particularly in children. The clinical phenomenology may mimic dopa-responsive dystonia (DRD) syndromes when NMDARE presents with oculogyric crises which is common in some DRDs.[7] Mitochondrial disorders in children may also present with dystonia and encephalopathy.

Myoclonus

Myoclonus, particularly when it presents in a subacute manner with coexisting encephalopathy, should raise suspicion of acquired entities such as autoimmune encephalopathies, infections (prion disease and Whipple disease), and metabolic derangements (uremia and liver failure), most of which are treatable. Predominant orthostatic leg myoclonus is a characteristic phenotype associated with contactin-associated protein-like 2 (CASPR2) antibody-mediated autoimmune disorders.[7] Myoclonus is also a defining feature of opsoclonus-myoclonus-ataxia syndrome (OMAS), frequently associated with neuroblastoma in children. Paraneoplastic OMAS in adults is associated with breast and lung cancer.[7]

Chorea

Immune-mediated conditions need to be considered when chorea occurs acutely or subacutely both in children and in adults. SC, discussed above, is the classical immune-mediated choreatic disorder in children. Other immune choreatic disorders to be considered in adults include the APLA syndrome and rarer conditions such as anti-Hu, anti-collapsin response-mediator protein-5 (CRMP5), anti-phosphodiesterase 10A (PDE10A) and anti-neurexin-3α-related autoimmune encephalopathies. These are usually combined with additional neurological signs and symptoms and are often paraneoplastic in etiology **(Tables 2 and 3)**.[30]

TABLE 3: Differential diagnosis of autoimmune movement disorders (AMDs) based on each movement disorder phenomenology.

Movement disorder phenomenology	Target antigens of the associated autoantibodies
Chorea/unclassified dyskinesias[2,31]	CV2/CRMP5, Hu, CASPR2, LGI1, NMDAR, Neurexin-3α, GABAAR, Dopamine-2-R, IgLON5, and PDE10A
Dystonia [2,31]	NMDAR, LGI1, Ri, Dopamine-2-R, IgLON5, CV2/CRMP5, Ma2, and GABAAR
Myoclonus	CASPR2, LGI1, DPPX, Neurexin-3α, and GlyR
Opsoclonus–myoclonus syndrome	VGCC, NMDAR, DPPX, GABAAR, GABABR, GlyR, GAD, CV2/CRMP5, Hu, Ri, Ma2, Zic4, and Yo
Tremor	CASPR2, LGI1, NMDAR, DPPX, GFAP, and Yo
Myorhythmia	IgLON5 and NMDAR
Stiff-person syndrome	GAD, GlyR, Amphiphysin, Gephyrin, DPPX, GABAAR, and Ri
PERM	GlyR, GAD, and DPPX
Parkinsonism	Ma2, IgLON5, Dopamine-2-R, DPPX, LGI1, Ri, CV2/CRMP5, and NMDARE
Ataxia	CASPR2, DPPX, NMDAR, IgLON5, VGCC, mGluR1, GAD, Yo, Hu, Ri, PCA2, Zic4, SOX1, and GFAP
Sleep-related movement disorders	IgLON5, Ma, LGI1, NMDAR, DPPX, CASPR2, and GABABR

(AQP4: aquaporin-4; CASPR2: contactin-associated protein-like 2; CV2/CRMP5: collapsin response-mediator protein 5; DPPX: dipeptidylpeptidase-like protein-6; GABAAR: γ-aminobutyric acid A receptor; GABABR: γ-aminobutyric acid B receptor; GAD: glutamic acid decarboxylase; GFAP: glial fibrillary acidic protein; GlyR: glycine receptor; IgLON5: immunoglobulin-like cell adhesion molecule 5; LGI1: leucine-rich glioma-inactivated 1; mGLuR1: metabotropic glutamate receptor type 1; mGLuR5: metabotropic glutamate receptor type 5; NMDARE: N-methyl-D-aspartate receptor encephalitis; PCA2: Pürkinje cell antibody 2; PDE10A: phosphodiesterase 10A; VGCC: voltage-gated calcium channel; Zic4: zinc finger domain of the intracellular transcription factor)

Peripheral Nerve Hyperexcitability and Related Conditions

Neuromyotonia (Issac syndrome) is a peripheral nerve hyperexcitability disorder clinically characterized by continuous muscle activity and manifesting as muscle stiffness, cramps, and myokymia. Morvan syndrome is a more severe condition with peripheral nerve hyperexcitability associated with myoclonus, encephalopathy, insomnia, neuromyotonia, and dysautonomia, seen in LGI-1 or CASPR2-related disorders.[31]

Stiff-person syndrome (SPS) is a clinical diagnosis characterized by fluctuating trunk and proximal limb (predominantly legs) rigidity, superimposed spasms, and exaggerated startle response (hyperekplexia), supported by the presence of autoantibodies.[7,32] Painful spasms are provoked by loud noise, touch, emotion, and stress, and are relieved dramatically with diazepam.[28,31] The presence of SPS, especially among females aged 40–60 years, should trigger a search for antibodies against glutamic acid decarboxylase (GAD), amphiphysin, gephyrin, glycine receptor (GlyR), dipeptidyl peptidase-like protein-6 (DPPX), and γ-aminobutyric acid A receptor (GABAAR).[7] Paraneoplastic SPS associated with anti-amphiphysin antibodies affects the older population, has a predilection for the upper limbs and neck region, and may be associated with myelopathy and sensory neuropathy.[7,28] Progressive encephalomyelitis with rigidity and myoclonus (PERM) is more often seen with GlyR antibodies and has an aggressive course with brainstem and autonomic dysfunction and long-tract signs.[8,28]

Other Movement Disorders

Tics form part of the clinical spectrum of PANDAS.[7] There have been unresolved debates on the epidemiology and pathophysiology of this entity and there are no evidence-based treatment recommendations. There are also certain sleep-related movement disorders described in autoimmune disorders affecting the CNS. Examples include status dissociatus (disintegration of stages of sleep boundaries with motor hyperactivity) and agrypnia excitata (insomnia, motor, and autonomic hyperactivity), which are seen in Morvan syndrome with anti-CASPR2,[30] and some other autoimmune encephalopathies.

The AMDs to be suspected based on a particular phenomenology are outlined in **Table 3**.

Knowledge regarding the distinct phenotypes and high index of suspicion is essential for diagnosing AMD and early initiation of immunotherapy.

Investigations in Suspected Autoimmune Movement Disorders

The investigations suggested for the workup of AMDs include MRI of the brain, CSF study, EEG, investigations like imaging studies, histopathology and tumor markers for underlying malignancy, and specific autoantibody testing. The positive findings favoring a diagnosis of AMD are mainly related to signs of inflammation in CSF (pleocytosis, elevated protein, IgG index, and oligoclonal bands) and MRI brain (T2 hyperintensities and gadolinium enhancement). **Figures 1 and 2** demonstrate representative MR images in selected AMDs.

There are various laboratory methods available for testing for autoantibodies. Western blot, indirect immunofluorescence (IFA), and immunohistochemistry (IHC) are essentially screening tests. To increase the specificity in the case of atypical clinical phenotypes, cell-based assays (CBA) are also recommended.[7] The interpretation of antibody testing results differs depending on the sample used. Antibodies to aquaporin P4 (AQP4) or voltage-gated potassium channels

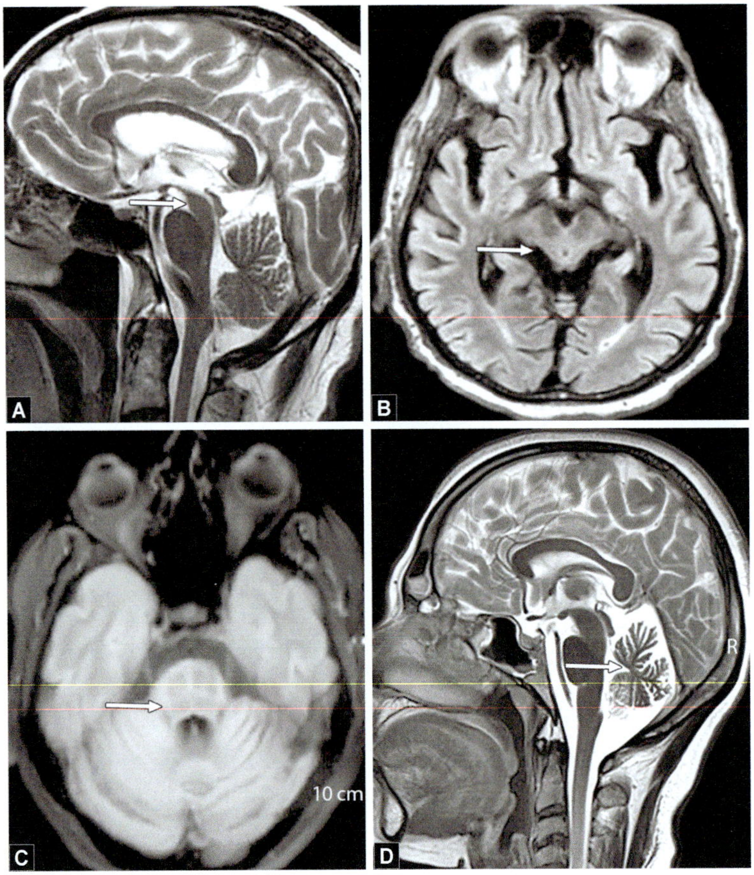

FIGS. 1A TO D: Magnetic resonance imaging (MRI) of the brain in autoimmune movement disorders. (A and B) Show T2-weighted sagittal and axial fluid-attenuated inversion recovery (FLAIR) sequences from a 54-year-old gentleman who presented with subacute onset axial parkinsonism from anti-immunoglobulin-like cell adhesion molecule family member 5 (IgLON5) antibody-related disease. The images show midbrain atrophy. (C) is the axial FLAIR image from a 62-year-old lady who presented with progressive ataxia, sleep dysfunction, and subtle parkinsonism. Cerebrospinal fluid (CSF) anti-IgLON5 antibodies were positive. The image shows "hot-cross-bun sign". (D) Shows T2-weighted sagittal image of the brain of a 50-year-old lady with anti-Yo encephalitis. The image shows significant cerebellar vermian atrophy.

(VGKC) are readily detected in serum, whereas others like anti-NMDAR or anti-GlyR are more relevant when demonstrated in CSF.[33] This could be largely due to technical factors leading to easier detection of these antibodies in CSF compared to serum or due to intrathecal antibody synthesis.[7] Overall, sensitivity and specificity are highest when both serum and CSF are tested **(Table 3)**.

SERONEGATIVE AUTOIMMUNE MOVEMENT DISORDER

Newer antibodies are being constantly added to the group of autoantibodies associated with neurological disorders every year, and hence it is obvious that there could be "antibody-negative" cases of autoimmune neurological disorders whose immunopathology is yet to

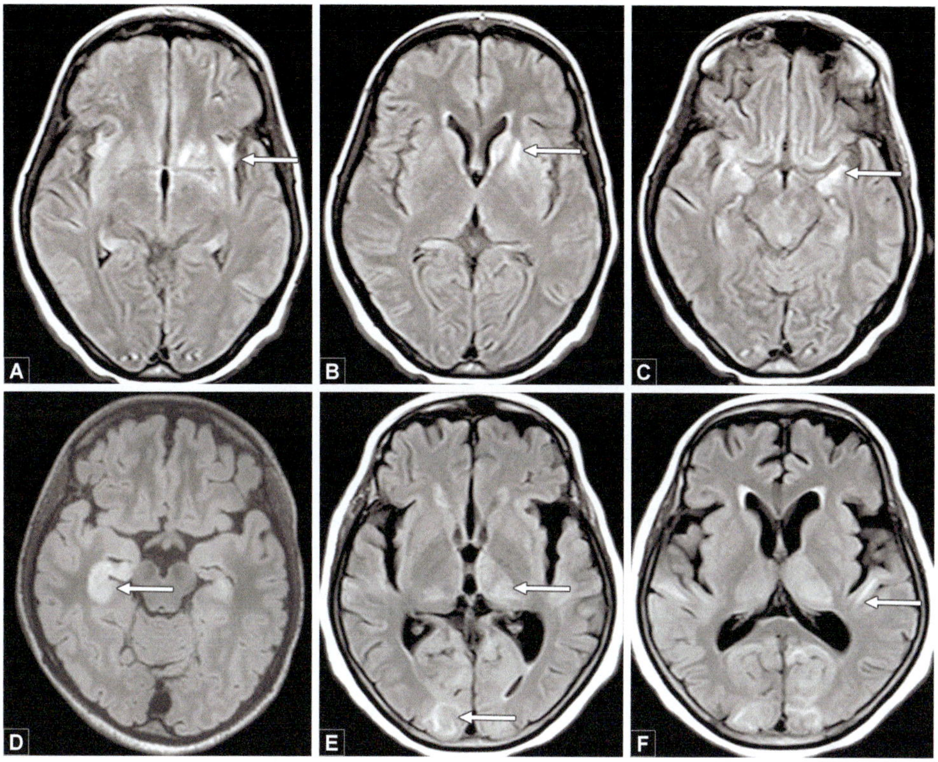

FIGS. 2A TO F: The images in the upper panel (A to C) show axial fluid-attenuated inversion recovery (FLAIR) sequences from a 50-year-old lady who presented with subacute onset encephalopathy and generalized dystonia. The images show hyperintensities in the basal ganglia, insula, and medial temporal lobes. Antibody testing was negative and the patient responded to immunotherapy. (D) Shows bilateral hippocampal hyperintensity in axial FLAIR sequences, in a 35-year-old lady with limbic encephalitis who was also antibody-negative. (E and F) Show multiple thalamic, cortical, and subcortical hyperintensities in a 72-year-old lady with anti-Ri encephalitis (arrows).

be discovered. Increased awareness regarding autoimmune neurological disorders has led to an increase in the diagnosis and sometimes overdiagnosis of AMDs in seronegative patients. The most important reasons for misdiagnosis include nonadherence to diagnostic criteria (particularly, exclusion of alternate diagnosis), failure to look for and give weightage to inflammatory changes in CSF and MRI, and limited use or unavailability of antibody testing.[34] Considering the treatability factor, the clinician is often biased toward making a diagnosis of seronegative AMD without adequate workup. When deciding the management strategy in seronegative AMDs, the treating physician needs to judiciously weigh the potential toxicity of the available immunotherapy options against the treatability factor, likelihood of an autoimmune etiology for the neurological syndrome in question, and chances of a progressive downhill course if immunotherapy is not administered **(Flowchart 1)**. Guidelines have been proposed to diagnose autoimmune encephalopathies when testing shows no autoantibodies.[34] These could be adapted to make a diagnosis of seronegative AMDs.

Step 1: Identify the phenomenology of the movement disorder (Dystonia, chorea, myoclonus, etc., or mixed)
Clues for autoimmune etiology: Acute or subacute onset; rapid progression; mixed movement disorders, accompanied by cognitive decline, seizures, presence of malignancy

↓

Step 2: Fit into a syndrome (e.g., Limbic encephalitis syndrome, anti-NMDARE syndrome) based on clinical phenomenology, whenever possible, and test for associated antibodies. If not fit with any specific syndrome, order for broader panels of antibodies associated with autoimmune encephalitis and paraneoplastic neurological syndromes. Look for evidence of neuro-inflammation in CSF and MRI. Workup for underlying malignancies based on the clinical syndrome and/or antibody detected

↓

Step 3: Treatment: Immunotherapy; tumor removal, whenever detected; symptomatic treatment for the movement disorder, based on clinical phenomenology

↓

Step 4: Immunotherapy for seronegative AMDs: The decision is to be individualized, based on the presence of typical clinical syndrome; subacute onset and progression; exclusion of other causes, and paraclinical evidence of neuroinflammation

FLOWCHART 1: Algorithm for evaluation and management of suspected autoimmune movement disorder (AMD).

(CSF: cerebrospinal fluid; NMDARE: N-methyl-D-aspartate receptor encephalitis)

The following features should lead to a high index of suspicion for AMDs even when antibody testing is negative:

- Rapid progression (<3 months) of the movement disorder with or without working memory deficits, altered mental status, and psychiatric symptoms.
- At least two of the following features suggesting inflammation of the brain: (1) MRI abnormalities suggesting AIE, (2) CSF pleocytosis, CSF-specific oligoclonal bands, or elevated CSF IgG index in the absence of any infection, and (3) brain biopsy showing inflammatory infiltrates.
- Reasonable exclusion of alternative causes

Alternative diagnoses to be excluded in patients with symptoms suggestive of AMDs include, but are not limited to the following: CNS infections (Herpes simplex encephalitis, Japanese encephalitis, neurosyphilis), Whipple disease, human immunodeficiency virus (HIV), Creutzfeldt-Jakob disease, septic encephalopathy, metabolic encephalopathy (uremia, liver failure, carbon monoxide poisoning, etc.), drug toxicity, Reye syndrome, "brain fog" (deficits in memory, attention, and executive functions) occurring as a result of chemotherapy, polypharmacy, or postcoronavirus disease (COVID), first onset psychosis and psychiatric disorders, functional movement disorders, epileptic disorders, mitochondrial diseases and neurometabolic disorders, neoplastic disorders (mainly glioma and lymphoma), vasculitis of CNS and rapidly progressive neurodegenerative or genetic disorders.

PRINCIPLES OF MANAGEMENT

Symptomatic treatment of movement disorders in autoimmune neurological syndromes is summarized in **Table 4**. The symptomatic treatment of movement disorders should be accompanied by correcting the metabolic derangements, such

TABLE 4: Symptomatic treatment offered for movement disorders.

Movement disorder phenomenology	Pharmacotherapy options
Dystonia	Anticholinergics, benzodiazepines, baclofen, tetrabenazine, and botulinum toxin injections
Chorea	Tetrabenazine, typical and atypical antipsychotics, benzodiazepines, amantadine, and anticonvulsants (sodium valproate particularly for rheumatic chorea)
Myoclonus	Benzodiazepines, sodium valproate, and levetiracetam
Tics	Tetrabenazine, clonidine, antipsychotics, and benzodiazepines
Tremor	Levodopa and dopamine agonists (Parkinsonian tremor and/or Holmes tremor), anticholinergics, botulinum toxin injections (dystonic tremor), propranolol, and clonazepam
Parkinsonism	Levodopa, dopamine agonists, and amantadine

as rhabdomyolysis or acute respiratory failure, secondary to severe movement disorders.[29] Mechanical ventilation may be needed when intravenous (IV) sedating medications or anesthetics are used for refractory and severe movement disorders like status dystonicus.

Immunotherapy must be initiated as early as possible, once the diagnosis is made. The response to immunotherapy depends on the type of antibody, with those targeting cell-surface antigens having a more favorable outcome compared to diseases associated with intracellular antibodies. The first-line therapy in most conditions is IV methylprednisolone at a dosage of 1 g for 3–5 days, followed by oral prednisolone, IVIG at a dosage of 0.4 g/kg for 5 days, and/or plasmapheresis (40–60 mL/kg) administered on alternate days for 10–14 days.[35]

If the patient is refractory to first-line treatment, second-line therapy should be considered without delay. Anti-CD20 therapy with rituximab (375 mg/m^2 weekly for 4 weeks or two doses of 750 mg/m^2, 2 weeks apart) or IV cyclophosphamide (750–1,000 mg/m^2 monthly for 3–6 months) are the most widely prescribed second-line agents.[35] Long-term maintenance therapy, with agents like low-dose prednisolone or other steroid-sparing medications (e.g., azathioprine or mycophenolate mofetil), should be considered for patients whose diseases relapse or who respond poorly to other medications.[35] Methotrexate, oral cyclophosphamide, and hydroxychloroquine are some of the alternatives.[35] It should be remembered that most of these drugs are associated with significant toxicity and major adverse effects profile and the patients should be closely monitored for the same.

Careful examination and investigations for a paraneoplastic etiology and prompt treatment of the underlying malignancy whenever detected, with surgery, radiotherapy, chemotherapy, or other targeted treatments as per standard recommendations, are crucial from both neurological and oncological point of view, for a better outcome. The development of new movement disorders in a patient previously treated for malignancy could indicate a tumor recurrence.[36]

CONCLUSION

Identification of autoimmune etiology in movement disorders is important as most of these syndromes are responsive to early immunotherapy, with some even achieving complete remission. A careful analysis of clinical features including movement disorder phenomenology guides antibody testing. The presence of characteristic clinical syndromes, acute or subacute presentation, and evidence for inflammation of neuroparenchyma in ancillary investigations can help to ascertain autoimmune etiology even when antibody testing is negative. Treatment of AMDs with immunotherapy is largely empirical and based on expert consensus opinion, rather than on evidence from randomized-controlled trials. Immunotherapy is potentially toxic and hence a careful weighing of the likelihood of autoimmune etiology from clinical features and investigations, against the potential toxicity of treatment options should be done in individual cases, particularly when antibody testing is negative and the clinical syndrome is not typical of AMD.

REFERENCES

1. Dutt M, Hallman-Cooper J, Bery E, Shahnawaz M, Gombolay G. Autoimmune Movement Disorders in Children: A Clinical Approach. Pract Neurol. 2020;34-40.
2. Hsieh PC, Wu YR. Diagnosis and Clinical Features in Autoimmune-Mediated Movement Disorders. J Mov Disord. 2022;15(2):95-105.
3. Graus F, Titulaer MJ, Balu R, Benseler S, Bien CG, Cellucci T, et al. A clinical approach to diagnosis of autoimmune encephalitis. Lancet Neurol. 2016;15(4):391-404.
4. Graus F, Vogrig A, Muñiz-Castrillo S, Antoine JCG, Desestret V, Dubey D, et al. Updated Diagnostic Criteria for Paraneoplastic Neurologic Syndromes. Neurol Neuroimmunol Neuroinflammation. 2021;8(4):e1014.
5. Menozzi E, Mulroy E, Akbarian-Tefaghi L, Bhatia KP, Balint B. Movement disorders in systemic autoimmune diseases: Clinical spectrum, ancillary investigations, pathophysiological considerations. Parkinsonism Relat Disord. 2021;88:116-28.
6. Dalmau J, Geis C, Graus F. Autoantibodies to Synaptic Receptors and Neuronal Cell Surface Proteins in Autoimmune Diseases of the Central Nervous System. Physiol Rev. 2017;97(2):839-87.
7. Balint B, Vincent A, Meinck HM, Irani SR, Bhatia KP. Movement disorders with neuronal antibodies: syndromic approach, genetic parallels and pathophysiology. Brain. 2018;141(1):13-36.
8. Mohammad SS, Ramanathan S, Brilot F, Dale RC. Autoantibody-associated movement disorders. Neuropediatrics. 2013;44(6):336-45.
9. Binks S, Uy C, Honnorat J, Irani SR. Paraneoplastic neurological syndromes: a practical approach to diagnosis and management. Pract Neurol. 2022;22(1):19-31.
10. Gable MS, Sheriff H, Dalmau J, Tilley DH, Glaser CA. The frequency of autoimmune N-methyl-D-aspartate receptor encephalitis surpasses that of individual viral etiologies in young individuals enrolled in the California Encephalitis Project. Clin Infect Dis. 2012;54(7):899-904.
11. Balint B, Bhatia KP. Autoimmune movement disorders with neuronal antibodies—an update. Curr Opin Neurol. 2021;34(4):565.
12. Dalmau J, Armangué T, Planagumà J, Radosevic M, Mannara F, Leypoldt F, et al. An update on anti-NMDA receptor encephalitis for neurologists and psychiatrists: mechanisms and models. Lancet Neurol. 2019;18(11):1045-57.
13. Vijayaraghavan A, Sundaram S, Sachithanandan S, Sukumaran S. Gyratory Seizures: An Early Clue to Anti-NMDAR Encephalitis. Indian J Pediatr. 2023;90(6):622.
14. Balu R, McCracken L, Lancaster E, Graus F, Dalmau J, Titulaer MJ. A score that predicts 1-year functional status in patients with anti-NMDA receptor encephalitis. Neurology. 2019;92(3):e244-52.
15. Gresa-Arribas N, Planagumà J, Petit-Pedrol M, Kawachi I, Katada S, Glaser CA, et al. Human neurexin-3α antibodies associate with encephalitis and alter synapse development. Neurology. 2016;86(24):2235-42.
16. Sabater L, Gaig C, Gelpi E, Bataller L, Lewerenz J, Torres-Vega E, et al. A novel non-rapid-eye movement and rapid-eye-movement parasomnia with sleep breathing disorder associated with antibodies to IgLON5: a case series, characterisation of the antigen, and post-mortem study. Lancet Neurol. 2014;13(6):575-86.
17. Grüter T, Möllers FE, Tietz A, Dargvainiene J, Melzer N, Heidbreder A, et al. Clinical, serological and genetic predictors of response to immunotherapy in anti-IgLON5 disease. Brain. 2023;146(2):600-11.
18. Nogueras-Ortiz CJ, De Jesús-Cortes HJ, Vaquer-Alicea J, Vega IE. Novel autoimmune response in a tauopathy mouse model. Front Neurosci. 2014;7:277.

19. Madetko N, Marzec W, Kowalska A, Przewodowska D, Alster P, Koziorowski D. Anti-IgLON5 Disease—The Current State of Knowledge and Further Perspectives. Front Immunol. 2022;13:852215.
20. Gaig C, Sabater L. New knowledge on anti-IgLON5 disease. Curr Opin Neurol. 2024;37(3):316.
21. Dalmau J, Graus F, Villarejo A, Posner JB, Blumenthal D, Thiessen B, et al. Clinical analysis of anti-Ma2-associated encephalitis. Brain. 2004;127(8):1831-44.
22. Yamamoto T, Tsuji S. Anti-Ma2-associated encephalitis and paraneoplastic limbic encephalitis. Brain Nerve. 2010;62(8):838-51.
23. Zuliani L, Sabater L, Saiz A, Baiges JJ, Giometto B, Graus F. Homer 3 autoimmunity in subacute idiopathic cerebellar ataxia. Neurology. 2007;68(3):239-40.
24. Mulroy E, Balint B, Bhatia KP. Homer-3 Antibody Disease: A Potentially Treatable MSA-C Mimic. Mov Disord Clin Pract. 2022;9(2):178-82.
25. Mandel-Brehm C, Dubey D, Kryzer Thomas J, O'Donovan Brian D, Tran B, Vazquez Sara E, et al. Kelch-like Protein 11 Antibodies in Seminoma-Associated Paraneoplastic Encephalitis. N Engl J Med. 2019;381(1):47-54.
26. Gyongyosi B, Magyar-Stang R, Takacs T, Szekely E, Illes Z, Nilsson C, et al. Paraneoplastic Kelch-like protein 11 antibody-associated cerebellar and limbic encephalitis caused by metastatic "burned-out" seminoma - A scar(r)y phenomenon. J Neuroimmunol. 2023;378:578073.
27. Vogrig A, Péricart S, Pinto AL, Rogemond V, Muñiz-Castrillo S, Picard G, et al. Immunopathogenesis and proposed clinical score for identifying Kelch-like protein-11 encephalitis. Brain Commun. 2021;3(3):fcab185.
28. Baizabal-Carvallo JF, Jankovic J. Movement disorders in autoimmune diseases. Mov Disord. 2012;27(8):935-46.
29. Nair SK. Autoimmune Movement Disorders. In: Ranganathan LN, Krishnan M, Iyer RS (Eds). Monograph: Immune-mediated neurological disorders. New Delhi: Jaypee Brothers Medical Publishers (P) Ltd.; 2022. pp. 67-75.
30. Balint B. Autoimmune Movement Disorders in Adults. Pract Neurol. 2020;30-40.
31. Lim TT. Paraneoplastic autoimmune movement disorders. Parkinsonism Relat Disord. 2017;44:106-9.
32. Hadavi S, Noyce AJ, Leslie RD, Giovannoni G. Stiff person syndrome. Pract Neurol. 2011;11(5):272-82.
33. Mckeon A, Vincent A. Autoimmune movement disorders. Handb Clin Neurol. 2016;133:301-15.
34. Dalmau J, Graus F. Diagnostic criteria for autoimmune encephalitis: utility and pitfalls for antibody-negative disease. Lancet Neurol. 2023;22(6):529-40.
35. Honorat JA, McKeon A. Autoimmune Movement Disorders: a Clinical and Laboratory Approach. Curr Neurol Neurosci Rep. 2017;17(1):4.
36. Vijayaraghavan A, Alexander PT, Nair AV, Sivadasan A, Mani AM, Mathew D, et al. Clinical Spectrum, Therapeutic Outcomes and Prognostic predictors in Paraneoplastic Neurological Syndromes - Experiences from a Tertiary Care Center in India. Ann Indian Acad Neurol. 2021;24(1):32-9.
37. Stephen Benesh F. Trending Autoantibodies Causing Movement Disorders. Pract Neurol. 2020;70-3.
38. Deng B, Cai M, Qiu Y, Liu X, Yu H, Zhang X, et al. MRI Characteristics of Autoimmune Encephalitis With Autoantibodies to GABAA Receptor: A Case Series. Neurol Neuroimmunol Neuroinflammation. 2022;9(3):e1158.
39. Boronat A, Sabater L, Saiz A, Dalmau J, Graus F. GABAB receptor antibodies in limbic encephalitis and anti-GAD–associated neurologic disorders. Neurology. 2011;76(9):795-800.
40. Dale RC, Merheb V, Pillai S, Wang D, Cantrill L, Murphy TK, et al. Antibodies to surface dopamine-2 receptor in autoimmune movement and psychiatric disorders. Brain. 2012;135(11):3453-68.
41. Fang B, McKeon A, Hinson SR, Kryzer TJ, Pittock SJ, Aksamit AJ, et al. Autoimmune Glial Fibrillary Acidic Protein Astrocytopathy: A Novel Meningoencephalomyelitis. JAMA Neurol. 2016;73(11):1297-307.
42. Wang S, Hou H, Tang Y, Zhang S, Wang G, Guo Z, et al. An overview on CV2/CRMP5 antibody-associated paraneoplastic neurological syndromes. Neural Regen Res. 2023;18(11):2357-64.

CHAPTER 12

Movement Disorders in the Emergency Room

Sreenivas UM, Lakshmanan S

ABSTRACT

"Movement Disorders" in the emergency room represent a group of conditions where urgent recognition and management are necessary and can be potentially reversible. Phenotype recognition is the first step, with differentiation between hypo- and hyperkinetic movement disorder. A thorough analysis of underlying cause and precipitating factors, including medication and infections, is needed as well. There are other emergencies, where there can be acute worsening of an underlying condition, or a new nonmotor complication of the movement disorder, such as laryngeal stridor in multiple system atrophy (MSA). Keen observation is important, since there are certain phenomenologies, which are characteristics of the underlying condition. In the correct clinical setting, this can expedite diagnosis and proper management. Supportive care is the first line of management, where intensive care and stabilization will be necessary. Mortality usually occurs due to renal failure following rhabdomyolysis or respiratory failure due to laryngeal or respiratory muscle involvement.

Keywords: Neuroleptic malignant syndrome, Acute parkinsonism, Status dystonicus, Status myoclonus, Choreic status, Serotonin syndrome, Catatonia.

INTRODUCTION

The general perception of "Movement Disorders" is of diseases with either degenerative or genetic etiologies, with treatable conditions being few and far in between. In the majority of clinical practice, this holds true. However, the emergency room is the one place where movement disorders are much more likely to be treatable and rapidly reversible.

The presentation of movement disorder as an emergency can be classified into two groups:

1. Acute movement disorder presentation of a systemic condition
2. Acute worsening of an underlying "Movement Disorder"

In this chapter, we will look at how to approach movement disorders in the emergency room, with diagnostic clues, urgent investigations, and possible therapeutic options.

APPROACH

The approach to diagnosing movement disorder emergencies remains the same as any other movement disorder. There are three steps to identifying the etiology:

1. The first step remains identifying the primary phenomenology.

2. The second step is to identify the movement disorder syndrome, by taking into account all the other phenomenologies seen, along with other neurological findings.
3. The third step is to analyze the possible etiologies, which can cause the specific syndrome which has been identified.

The phenomenologies are classified into hypokinetic or hyperkinetic movement disorders.[1] The hypokinetic movement disorder emergencies encountered are:

- *Akinetic rigid syndromes*:
  - Neuroleptic malignant syndrome
  - Serotonin syndrome
  - Parkinson-hyperpyrexia syndrome
  - Acute parkinsonism
- *Catatonia*:
  - Malignant catatonia
- *Stiffness*:
  - Status spasticus in Stiff person spectrum disorder

The hyperkinetic movement disorder emergencies are:

- *Dystonia*:
  - Dystonic storm
  - Acute dystonic reaction
- *Myoclonus*:
  - Myoclonic status
  - Serotonin syndrome
- *Chorea*:
  - Choreic storm
- *Tic*:
  - Tic status
- Psychogenic movement disorders[1,2]

There is very little data on the prevalence or incidence of these conditions. A study from a tertiary care center in India reported that hyperkinetic movement disorders were much more likely to present as emergencies than hypokinetic. Among the hyperkinetic, chorea was the most common, followed by dystonia, myoclonus, and dyskinesia, in that order of prevalence. Among the etiologies recorded, hyperglycemia was the most common, followed by autoimmune, stroke, drug induced and infections. 10% did not have a clear etiology. The overall incidence of movement disorder emergencies was noted to be low at 0.2%.[3]

A similar study from Italy by Dallocchio et al. (2018) shows a similar incidence (0.073%), but found myoclonus to be the most common presentation, with drug induced being the most common etiology, probably reflecting cultural and ethnic differences in the population.[2,3]

Beyond these phenomenologies, there are syndromes where there are mixed phenomenologies, such as chorea, dystonia, and stereotypy, which can coexist in anti-N-methyl-D-aspartate receptor (NMDAR) encephalitis.

Emergencies can arise in patients with underlying movement disorders, such as:

- Acute laryngeal stridor in multiple system atrophy (MSA)
- Acute psychosis in Parkinson's disease or diffuse Lewy body disease
- Cervical myelopathy in severe cervical tics
- Severe self-harm in Tourette syndrome[3,4]

All etiologies of acute movement disorders can be classified into eight different groups:

1. Vascular
2. Infective
3. Trauma
4. Toxins
5. Autoimmune
6. Metabolic
7. Inflammation
8. Neoplastic

Hypokinetic emergencies:

- *Neuroleptic malignant syndrome*: It is known to occur following exposure to dopamine blockers. Typical antipsychotic has higher susceptibility (7.3%) compared to atypical antipsychotic (3.3%), as evidenced by haloperidol being the most common culprit.[1] Multiple dopamine blockers in combination have a higher risk compared to monotherapy. Concomitant use of lithium can precipitate the condition as well. Nonneuroleptic drugs can also produce a similar condition, termed "Neuroleptic malignant like syndrome".[1,2,4,5]

Drugs associated with the syndrome are listed in the **Table 1**.

Two-thirds of the cases of neuroleptic malignant syndrome present within 1 week of exposure to the drug, but the syndrome can manifest even months or years postexposure. The clinical tetrad manifests in the order of rigidity, hyperthermia, altered mental status followed by dysautonomia. Dystonia and tremors can also be seen. Dysautonomic features include tachycardia, labile blood pressure, profuse sweating, tachypnea, incontinence, etc. Altered mental status can worsen to mutism, catatonia, and even coma.

- *Serotonin syndrome*: This syndrome is driven by excess serotonergic activity in the nervous system, unlike neuroleptic malignant syndrome or parkinsonism-hyperpyrexia syndrome (PHS). Data on the syndrome is scarce and the incidence is 0.5–0.9/1,000 cases on selective serotonin reuptake inhibitor (SSRI) monotherapy as per the United Kingdom (UK) study. SSRI overdose (14–16%) is the most common cause along with multiple drug combinations, especially SSRI and monoamine oxidase (MAO) inhibitors.[1] Drugs causing the syndrome are listed in **Table 2**.

TABLE 1: Drugs causing neuroleptic malignant syndrome.

Class	Drugs
Psychiatric	Risperidone, ziprasidone, haloperidol, clozapine, loxapine, chlorpromazine, fluphenazine, thiothixene, olanzapine, and thioridazine
Antiemetics	Prochlorperazine and promethazine
Properistaltic	Metoclopramide, domperidone, levosulpiride, itopride, and cisapride
Antiparkinsonian	Levodopa and dopamine agonists

TABLE 2: Drugs associated with serotonin syndrome.

Drugs	Examples
Selective serotonin reuptake inhibitors (SSRIs) and selective serotonin and norepinephrine reuptake inhibitors (SNRIs)	• Sertraline • Paroxetine • Fluoxetine • Citalopram • Escitalopram • Venlafaxine • Desvenlafaxine • Duloxetine
Monoamine oxidase inhibitors	• Amitriptyline • Nortriptyline • Clomipramine • Imipramine
Other psychiatropics	• Lithium • Trazodone • Bupropion
Recreational and "street" drugs	• Cocaine • "Ecstasy" (MDMA) • Lysergic acid diethylamide (LSD)
Antiepileptic	Valproic acid
Antibiotics and antiviral	• Linezolid • Ritonavir
Cough and cold	Dextromethorphan
Analgesics and relaxants	• Tramadol • Fentanyl • Meperidine • Cyclobenzaprine
Dietary supplements	• Ginseng • St. John's wort • Tryptophan
Antiemetic and properistaltic	• Ondansetron • Metoclopramide

Serotonin syndrome is a close mimic of other akinetic rigid syndromes, such as neuroleptic malignant syndrome, but can be differentiated by the presence of myoclonus, seizures, hypereflexia, ataxia, diarrhea, and profuse sweating.[1,2,4]

- *Malignant catatonia*: This is a life-threatening manifestation of catatonia, commonly in a patient with preexisting psychiatric illness. Patients present with profound behavior change, followed by severe akinesia. The clinical manifestation can be divided into three phases; prodromal phase, severe motor excitement phase, and the final phase:
    1. *Prodromal phase*: This is the period of profound altered behavior with anxiety, insomnia, agitation, etc. This can last up to 2 weeks.
    2. *Severe motor excitement phase*: This phase is characterized by altered mental status, rigidity, and dysautonomia. There can be periodic exacerbations of the symptoms as well.
    3. *Final phase*: This phase has extreme hyperthermia and cardiovascular collapse, which can lead to stupor and coma.[1,2,4,6,7]
- *Parkinson-hyperpyrexia syndrome*: This is a neuroleptic malignant syndrome like clinical picture, seen in patients with Parkinson's disease. This is usually seen on reduction of dose or withdrawal of dopaminergic drugs. Patients classically present with akinesia, increased tone, hyperthermia, etc., mimicking neuroleptic malignant syndrome. In comparison to other hypokinetic emergencies, this syndrome has profound extrapyramidal features namely rigidity, tremor, akinesia, and bradykinesia. These symptoms are accompanied by hyperthermia and autonomic dysfunction in rare cases. The symptoms can set in up to 7 days after the withdrawal of the drug. Dehydration, infection, and metabolic conditions can also precipitate the condition. A rare etiology of this syndrome is the failure of a deep brain stimulation (DBS) system.[1,2,4,6,7]
- *Acute parkinsonism*: In general, Parkinsonism has a gradual onset, slow progress, and a chronic degenerative neurological course. In acute parkinsonism, the same condition arises in a rapid fashion over hours to weeks. The management of the condition solely depends upon the nature of the underlying cause. These causes are enumerated in **Table 3**.[1,2,4,6,7]
- *Status spasticus*: This is a rare but characteristic syndrome, where the presentation is presence of pain and paraspinal muscle spasms, which can last for days. This is seen as an acute worsening in patients with "Stiff-person Spectrum Disorder". Spasms can be spontaneous or brought about by noise or movement. Spinal cord compression can occur, but without symptomatic myelopathy. It can lead to fractures, joint subluxations, abdominal herniation, rhabdomyolysis and autonomic dysfunction, all of which can lead to severe morbidity or mortality.[6,8]

Hyperkinetic emergencies:

- *Chorea-ballismus*: Acute chorea can lead to hyperthermia and rhabdomyolysis. There are certain chorea syndromes which are characteristics of certain etiologies:
    - Childhood onset generalized chorea in the background of fever with joint pains—Sydenham's chorea. However, the chorea can develop months after the episode of rheumatic fever. Chorea usually resolves over time but can rarely become chronic or relapse later in life, especially during pregnancy.
    - *Generalized chorea in first trimester of pregnancy*: Chorea gravidarum. This is usually a relapse of Sydenham's chorea. Symptoms present within the first 12 weeks of pregnancy and resolve

TABLE 3: Causes of acute parkinsonism.

Drugs	Examples
Medications	• Prokinetics • Antipsychotics • SSRIs • Amphotericin-B • Chemotherapy • Immune checkpoint inhibitors
Toxins	• Carbon monoxide • Methanol • Cyanide • Organophosphate poisoning • MPTP
Structural brain lesions	• Basal ganglia and midbrain stroke • Pontine/Extrapontine myelinolysis • Hydrocephalus • Brainstem and posterior fossa tumors
Infectious and inflammatory conditions	• Systemic lupus erythematosus • Sarcoidosis • Brainstem encephalitis • Autoimmune or paraneoplastic encephalitis • Mycoplasma • HIV • Whipple disease
Neuropsychiatric	• Catatonia • Functional parkinsonism
Hereditary	• Wilson disease • Rapid onset dystonia parkinsonism

(HIV: human immunodeficiency virus; MPTP: 1-methyl-4-phenyl-1,2,3,6-tetrahydropyridine; SSRIs: selective serotonin reuptake inhibitors)

during pregnancy or immediately after birth.

- Generalized chorea, especially in women of child-bearing age—lupus and antiphospholipid antibody syndrome
- Hemiballismus—vascular insult to subthalamic nucleus
- *Hemiballismus,* especially in elderly females—nonketotic hyperglycemia (can be bilateral). This is a rare presentation with a worldwide prevalence of 1 in 100,000. However, it can also be the presenting symptom of diabetes mellitus. Usually, the chorea resolves with correction of the hyperglycemia. In 20%, it may persist for up to 3 months.
- *Generalized chorea in a patient with Parkinson's disease*: Levodopa induced dyskinesias and overactivity of DBS. This is particularly significant if the movements become continuous, and can lead to rhabdomyolysis. This can be triggered by infection, heat exposure, dehydration, dyselectrolytemia, or change in medication.
- Chorea in a middle-aged individual, especially if associated with altered behavior, seizures, and orofacial dyskinesias—autoimmune encephalitis, especially anti-NMDAR. Chorea can coexist with seizures, which can lead to underrecognition of the movement disorder.[6,7,9]

There are other causes of chorea which are tabulated in **Table 4**.

Dystonia

There are two different presentations of dystonia as an emergency:

1. *Dystonic storm*: Dystonic storm or status dystonicus is seen as an acute worsening of dystonia in patients who already have underlying generalized dystonic disorders of any etiology. There are severe and continuous contractures which can affect any part of the body, or can be generalized. The dystonia can be tonic (sustained) or phasic (rapid and repetitive). The episodes are associated with preserved consciousness, but the

TABLE 4: Causes of severe chorea.

Vascular	• Anoxia • Stroke: Ischemic/hemorrhagic • Vascular malformations • Polycythemia vera • Postcardiac bypass pump chorea • MELAS
Metabolic	• Nonketotic hyperglycemia • Hypoglycemia • Uremia • Hyperthyroidism • Hypoparathyroidism
Infectious	• Cryptococcosis • Toxoplasmosis • Tuberculoma • Mycoplasma • HIV encephalitis
Autoimmune	• Sydenham chorea • Systemic lupus erythematosus • Antiphospholipid antibody syndrome • Scleroderma • Behçet disease • Polyarteritis nodosa • Sarcoidosis • Multiple sclerosis • Paraneoplastic: CV2/CRMP5, NMDA, anti-Hu, anti-SOX, anti-PCA, anti-Yo, anti-Ri, and anti-Ma
Toxic	• Oral contraceptives • Levodopa • Cocaine • Amphetamine • Morphine • Methadone • Alcohol • Antiepileptics

(CRMP5: collapsin-response-mediator protein-5; HIV: human immunodeficiency virus; MELAS: mitochondrial encephalomyopathy with lactic acidosis and stroke-like episodes; NMDA: N-methyl-D-aspartate)

patient may be unable to communicate due to laryngeal or orofacial dystonia. Occasionally, respiratory muscles can be involved, leading to distress and urgent intubation. Prolonged dystonic storm can lead to rhabdomyolysis, renal failure, hyperthermia, and aspiration. Mortality is around 10%, occurring predominantly due to respiratory and renal failure.[5,7,9]

The cause of this worsening can be due to infections, trauma, or medication changes. It can also happen due to sudden failure of stimulation, if the patient already has DBS implanted. Other causes are listed in **Table 5**.

One of the emerging causes of acute dystonia is autoimmune/paraneoplastic

TABLE 5: Causes of dystonic storm.

Primary dystonia	• Rapid onset dystonia parkinsonism (DYT-12) • Infantile striatal necrosis • Wilson disease • Pantothenate kinase-associated neurodegeneration • Neuroacanthocytosis
Structural	• Traumatic brain injury • Stroke • Tumors • Birth injury • Inflammatory (MS and sarcoid) Tonic spasms in LETM
Toxic/ Iatrogenic	• Carbon monoxide poisoning • D2 antagonist use • ITB withdrawal
Metabolic	• Leigh disease • Aminoacidurias • Urea cycle disorders
Degenerative	Laryngeal spasm in MSA

(DYS-12: dystonia-12; ITB: intrathecal baclofen; LETM: longitudinally extensive transverse myelitis; MS: multiple sclerosis; MSA: multiple system atrophy)

encephalitis. There are specific phenomenologies, which can suggest an autoimmune etiology, such as:

- Faciobrachial dystonic jerks—seen in anti-LGI1 encephalitis
- Opisthotonus—seen in anti-NMDAR encephalitis
- Jaw dystonia and laryngospasm—seen in anti-Ri encephalitis[6,7,10]

2. *Acute dystonic reaction*: This is seen within 24 hours of exposure to dopamine receptor blockers, especially with more potent neuroleptics. It is reported to occur more frequently in men, especially when the drugs are titrated upward quickly. Manifestations depend on the body part involved, although there can be generalized dystonia as well.

   Some characteristic dystonic reactions are:

   - *Oculogyric crises*: The eyes have tonic upward deviation, along with retraction of eyelids, and occasionally retrocollis.
   - Spasmodic dysphonia—which can be life-threatening since breathing can be compromised.
   - Blepharospasm—classically seen with overactivity of the orbicularis oculi, which can involve either the pretarsal portion or the periorbital portion of the muscle, or both. Compensatory overactivity of the frontalis muscle can be seen (other Babinski sign).
   - Pisa syndrome or pleurothotonus—this is seen as abnormal sustained truncal posturing to one side.

Acute dystonic reactions can be seen with a wide variety of drugs. The most likely agents are haloperidol and fluphenazine. Other drugs reported to cause dystonic reaction are carbamazepine, methylphenidate, prokinetics, serotonergic drugs, and general anesthetics. In Wilson disease, use of penicillamine, zinc, or trientine can cause acute worsening. Use of metoclopramide can also cause this reaction, especially at doses above 30 mg. However, acute dystonic reaction can be idiosyncratic and nondose dependent, hence, it can develop in patients who have been taking dopamine blockers for a long time, without any obvious precipitant. Dehydration, dyselectrolytemia, and cocaine use increase the risk of dystonic reaction. This is also seen more commonly in younger age and in males. The overall incidence of acute dystonic reaction is only 1–2% of all patients exposed the drugs. Pisa syndrome can be triggered by neuroleptics, anticholinesterases, or can occur spontaneously in MSA and advanced Parkinson's disease.[1,4,7]

Myoclonus

Acute onset myoclonus usually suggests a metabolic derangement. This can be due to deranged electrolytes, kidney dysfunction, liver dysfunction or hypercarbia, or due to a drug intake. This is especially true if the myoclonus is predominantly negative. In renal failure or liver failure, the acuity of the insult, leading to rapid rise in urea levels, predisposed to myoclonus.

Multiple drugs have been reported to cause myoclonus, including serotonergic drugs, neuroleptics, opiates, antiepileptics (especially sodium channel inhibitors), propofol, calcium-channel blockers, gabapentin, antibiotics, and spinal anesthetics. These drugs are particularly prone to cause myoclonus if there is renal insufficiency.

In patients with Parkinson's disease, the development of acute myoclonus can indicate a few possibilities:

- Increase in levodopa dosage (especially levodopa-carbidopa intestinal gel)
- Depletion of vitamin B12
- Amantadine toxicity (which is usually triggered by renal impairment)

Myoclonus can also develop after hypoxia. Anoxic myoclonus can be of two types:

1. *Myoclonic status epilepticus*: Diffuse persistent myoclonus in comatose patients, which usually sets in hours after an anoxic insult. This is associated with a poor prognosis. Myoclonic status can also be seen.
2. *Lance-Adams syndrome*: This is characterized by stimulus sensitive and action induced myoclonus, which set in days after the anoxic insult. The course of the myoclonus can be variable and depends on severity of insult. Treatment may be necessary, if disabling.

Serotonin syndrome is a specific emergency where myoclonus is commonly seen. However, since patients are predominantly stiff in this condition, it is discussed under hypokinetic emergencies.

Opsoclonus-myoclonus syndrome or opsoclonus-myoclonus-ataxia syndrome is a condition where there can be acute onset generalized or multifocal myoclonus, in association with uncontrolled rapid eye movements, called opsoclonus. In many instances, patients are also unsteady and ataxic. This syndrome is commonly paraneoplastic and should prompt evaluation for underlying malignancy. Neuroblastoma remains the most commonly associated tumor in children. However, there are increasing reports of this syndrome as the presentation of viral encephalitis and Lyme disease.

While myoclonus, in general, is generalized, a unilateral myoclonus should raise suspicion of a structural lesion in the thalamus, of any etiology.[5-7]

Tics

There are two common emergency presentations of tics:

1. *Tic status*: This is an increase in severity and frequency of tics, leading to unremitting and self-injurious tics, which can interfere with her regular activities. Aggravation of tics is seen due to fatigue, stress, infection, and medications. Common drugs which can exacerbate tics are neurostimulants, SSRIs, and tricyclic antidepressants.
2. *Complication of tics*: Violent motor tics can lead to neurological complications. This occurs due to traumatic injury, leading to compressive cervical myelopathies, compressive neuropathies, subdural hematoma, etc.

Tics usually begin in childhood and may wax and wane into adulthood. Reemergence of childhood tics in adulthood is usually due to stress or drug use, such as neurostimulants.

Functional Movement Disorders

This is an extremely difficult diagnosis to make in the emergency room, since functional movement disorders can have any type of phenomenology. Many a time, functional tremors or hemifacial spasms can be mistaken for seizures. A newly emerging functional movement disorder is functional tic disorder, also called "tic-toc tics", which are emerging due to exposure to tics on social media.

Movement Disorder Mimics

There are certain conditions which can mimic a movement disorder, especially in an emergency. Early recognition is important since the treatment varies significantly. Some mimics are:

- *Limb shaking transient ischemic attack (TIAs)*: These are recurrent, brief, arrhythmic movements of one limb, usually seen in critical internal carotid artery stenosis, triggered by walking or standing. These movements can mimic hemichorea.
- *Epilepsia partialis continua*: These are focal motor seizures, which can be mistaken for tremors.

- *Retropharyngeal abscess, atlantoaxial subluxation*—both these conditions can mimic acute cervical dystonia. Pain is a useful clue to suspect these conditions.
- *Pseudoathetosis*—these are involuntary movements, which can mimic chorea. This is due to sensory ataxia, caused by either peripheral neuropathy or posterior column lesions.

DIAGNOSTIC CLUES

Autonomic instability, including hyperthermia, labile blood pressure, tachycardia, diaphoresis, etc., is seen in a few conditions:

- Neuroleptic malignant syndrome
- Serotonin syndrome
- Dystonic storm

The akinetic rigid syndromes—all attract attention for the marked paucity of movement noted. Among the hyperthermic akinetic rigid syndromes, there are certain similarities and differences. The differentiating features of each are shown in **Figure 1**.

The presence of hypotension on presentation, especially if associated with myoglobinuria, is suggestive of neuroleptic malignant syndrome or a dystonic storm.

Oculogyric crisis suggests either an acute dystonic reaction to medication or underlying disorder of dopamine synthesis pathway.

The presence of acute-to-subacute altered behavior, new onset seizures, when associated with a new onset movement disorder, especially if mixed, should raise the suspicion of an autoimmune encephalitis. There are specific phenotypes which should raise suspicion of specific antibody-mediated encephalitis:

- *Chorea*: NMDA, leucine-rich glioma-inactivated-1 (LGI1), contactin-associated protein-like 2 (CASPR2), gamma-aminobutyric acid $(GABA)_A$, $GABA_B$, D2, and

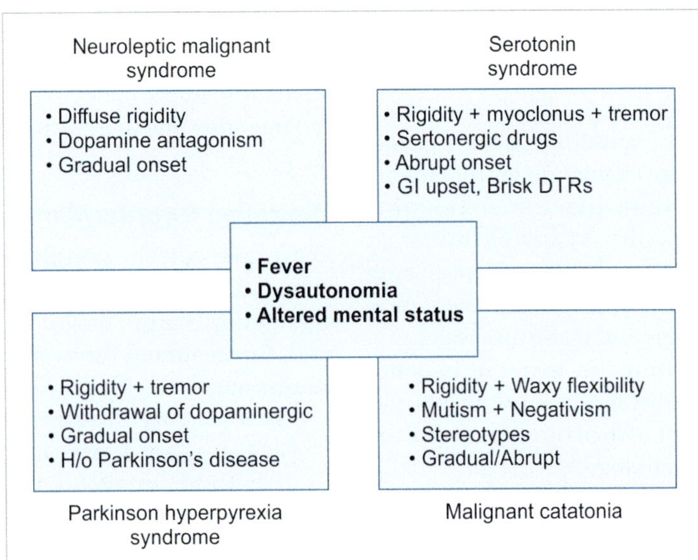

FIG. 1: The akinetic rigid syndrome.

(DTRs: deep tendon reflexes; GI: gastrointestinal; H/o: history of)

collapsin response-mediator protein-5 (CRMP-5)
- *Ataxia*: CASPR2, $GABA_B$, dipeptidyl-peptidase-like protein 6 (DPPX), D2, glutamic acid decarboxylase 65-kilodalton isoform (GAD65), CRMP5, glial fibrillary acidic protein (GFAP), and Ri
- *Opsoclonus myoclonus*: $GABA_A$, $GABA_B$, DPPX, CRMP5, Ri, and Ma2
- *Dystonia*: NMDA, LGI1 (facio-brachio dystonic seizures), D2, and Ri (jaw dystonia)
- *Orolingual dyskinesia*: NMDA and Neurexin-3α
- *Stiff-person syndrome*: $GABA_A$, DPPX, ampiphysin, and GAD65
- *Parkinsonism*: LGI1, D2, Ma2, and Ri[10]

Status spastics can be especially suspected if the patient has back muscles which are extremely hard on palpation, with a board-like appearance. Horizontal creases can be seen in the small of the back. Spasms can be brought on by auditory or tactile stimuli.[8]

There are certain clues which should raise suspicion of functional etiology:
- Fixed dystonia
- Unusual distribution which are incongruous with known syndromes
- Distractibility
- Entrainment
- Improvement with placebo/suggestion
- La belle indifference
- Bizarre gait
- Recent psychological trauma

Investigations

In the emergency room, the first investigation required is capillary blood glucose. The other important investigations are:
- Arterial blood glass—to look for metabolic acidosis and hypercarbia.
- Creatine phosphokinase—to monitor muscle overactivity and breakdown
- Serum urea, blood urea nitrogen (BUN), and creatinine—to identify early kidney dysfunction
- Urinalysis—to look for signs of infection, early kidney dysfunction or myoglobinuria
- Complete blood count—watch for signs of infection
- Blood cultures—to rule out underlying infections
- Electrolytes—identify hyperkalemia, and hypocalcemia which can result from rhabdomyolysis.

Specific tests for specific phenomenologies are:
- *Akinetic rigid syndromes*:
  - Creatine phosphokinase (CPK)—commonly elevated in majority of cases
  - Arterial blood gas (ABG)—to look for increasing lactate and metabolic acidosis
- *Chorea*:
  - In children—α-Streptolysin-O and anti-DNAse-B titers
  - In hemichorea—MRI to look for stroke/T1 hyperintensity of putamen in diabetic striatopathy, and capillary blood glucose levels
  - Acute generalized chorea—antiphospholipid antibody, anticardiolipin antibody, anti-β-2 glycoprotein antibody, and lupus anticoagulant
  - In generalized chorea, always rule out hyperthyroidism and electrolyte abnormalities, including calcium.
  - Complete blood count to look for polycythemia vera
  - Liver function tests and MRI imaging of brain to look for hepatocereberal degeneration
  - Serum ceruloplasmin, 24-hour urine copper—if Wilson disease is suspected.
- *Autoimmune encephalitis*:
  - Cerebrospinal fluid (CSF) analysis to look for elevated proteins
  - Cerebrospinal fluid cells to look for pleomorphic leukocytosis

- Whole body positron emission tomography (PET)/CT chest and abdomen to look for underlying malignancy
- Antibodies for specific antibodies. The choice of CSF or serum testing depends on specific syndrome being tested for:
  - Anti-NMDAR antibody is more sensitive in CSF.
  - Anti-LGI1 and anti-CASPR2 antibodies are more sensitive in the serum.

THERAPEUTIC OPTIONS

The approach to management of movement disorder emergencies is two pronged. Initial management focuses on stabilizing the patient and symptomatic management, followed by identification of the etiology and specific treatment.

Acute management also includes identifying precipitating factor, which might have triggered the emergency. This includes underlying systemic conditions such as:

- Hypo-/hyperglycemia
- Hypo-/hypernatermia
- Dehydration
- Depression
- Fever and/or sepsis
- Acute toxin ingestion
- Acute drug ingestion
- Change in drug regimen

There are some general rules which help in managing all movement disorder emergencies. These include:

- Ensure airway and breathing.
- Secure early intravenous (IV) access.
- Aggressive IV hydration (with caution if underlying heart disease)
- Early management of hyperthermia (seen in many movement disorder emergencies)
- Watch for autonomic instability.
- Intravenous sedation in severe disorders
- Investigate for dyselectrolytemia, organ dysfunction, and infections

Aggressive IV hydration helps to manage myoglobinuria and hypotension, as well as to correct the metabolic derangements which can occur in hyperkinetic emergencies. The continuous muscle activity leads to third spacing of fluids, causing hypovolemia and dyselectrolytemia. IV fluid replacement helps to reverse this complication.

Hyperthermia management can be either pharmacological, in the form of IV acetaminophen or nonsteroidal anti-inflammatory drugs (NSAIDs), or nonpharmacological such as cooling blankets. In extreme cases, where body temperature is above 40°C, more aggressive measures such as intravascular cooling catheters can be used. In such cases, continuous core temperature monitoring using esophageal probes is recommended.

Management of autonomic instability depends on early recognition of the components and addressing each individual component:

- Accelerated hypertension—managed by IV antihypertensives
- Hypotension—managed by IV vasopressors and hydration
- Labile blood pressure—requires continuous blood pressure monitoring with an arterial line
- Respiratory compromise—recognized by ABG monitoring for hypercarbia. The management is by endotracheal intubation and mechanical ventilatory support. In hyperkinetic emergencies, patients may require IV sedation or neuromuscular blockade, to facilitate intubation.

Disease-specific immediate management:

- *Acute dystonic reaction/ Dystonic status*:
  - Intravenous anticholinergics: diphenhydramine/benztropine, procyclidine 5-10 mg iv
  - Intravenous antihistamines
  - Benzodiazepines (BZDs)
  - Stereotactic surgery—including DBS

- *Choreic status*:
    - High potency neuroleptics
    - Tetrabenazine
    - Intravenous BZDs
    - Intravenous propofol
- *Myoclonic status*:
    - Valproate
    - Levetiracetam
    - Benzodiazepines
    - Deep brain stimulation—anoxic myoclonus
- *Tic status*:
    - High potency neuroleptics: Aripiprazole 5–15 mg/day
    - Tetrabenazine: 12.5–100 mg/day
    - Benzodiazepine
    - Clonidine
    - Botulinum toxin for focal tics
    - Deep brain stimulation in malignant Tourette syndrome
- *Neuroleptic malignant syndrome*:
    - Bromocriptine: 2.5 mg OD, up to 5 mg TDS
    - Amantadine: 100 mg OD to TDS
    - Dantrolene: 1–2.5 mg/kg IV q8h, up to 10 mg/kg/day
- *Serotonin syndrome*:
    - Cyproheptadine: 12 mg STAT, followed by 4–6 mg q6h, up to 32 mg/day
    - Propranolol
    - Vecuronium
    - Chlorpromazine: 50–100 mg intramuscularly (IM)
- *Malignant catatonia*:
    - Lorazepam: 1–2 g IM/IV q4–6 hours
    - Electroconvulsive therapy
- *Parkinson hyperpyrexia syndrome*:
    - Restart levodopa at premorbid dose
    - Ropinirole 1–2 mg TDS
    - Bromocriptine 5–10 mg/day in three divided doses
    - Subcutaneous apomorphine
    - Levodopa carbidopa intestinal gel
    - Methylprednisolone 1 g IV for 5 days
- *Acute parkinsonism*:
    - Levodopa trial
    - Dopa agonists to be avoided
    - IV methylprednisoloine, if chemotherapy induced/autoimmune
- *Status spasticus*:
    - Benzodiazepines—parenteral diazepam and oral clonazepam
    - Baclofen—oral at high doses/intrathecal
    - Tizanidine—2 mg TDS
    - Intravenous immunoglobulin—2 mg/kg over 5 days

Specific etiologies have specific medications which have better efficacy:

Chorea:

- *Sydenham chorea*: Valproic acid at doses of 10–25 mg/kg/day. Patients also need prolonged courses of penicillin to reduce risk of relapse. If prolonged and refractory, immunotherapy can be tried.
- *Hyperglycemic chorea*: Movements subside with control of blood sugars. Occasionally, they may persist for a few months and require additional medications such as dopamine receptor blockers, valproate, tetrabenazine, etc.
- *Chorea in systemic lupus erythematosus (SLE) or antiphospholipid antibody syndrome*: Movements respond to immunotherapy, such as pulse steroids, or if persistent, IV immunoglobulins can be tried.
- *Chorea gravidarum*: Usually, no treatment is given in 1st trimester. If chorea is severe and persistent, low dose of haloperidol can be tried in the 2nd trimester at doses of 0.5–2 mg, two to three times a day.

In "Dystonic Status", there are specific drugs which can be used to rapidly relieve symptoms:

- Enteral chloral hydrate 30–100 mg/kg q3–6 hourly—to achieve sleep

- Enteral or IV clonidine at high doses—acts as central nervous system (CNS) depressant
- Intravenous midazolam 30–100 μg/kg/hour
- Propofol 0.3–3 mg/kg/hour
- *Nondepolarizing paralytics*: Pancuronium/vecuronium

In cases of refractory to medications, other options include:

- Intrathecal baclofen, which can be a transition to a permanent baclofen pump.
- Deep brain stimulation of bilateral globus pallidus internus (GPi)
- Pallidotomy

In postanoxic myoclonus, there are a plethora of drugs which are useful.

- Clonazepam: 4–8 mg/day
- Valproate: 1,200–3,000 mg/day
- Levetiracetam: 1,000–3,000 mg/day
- Piracetam
- Perampanel

However, all of them have modest benefits. In rare cases of debilitating myoclonus, DBS of bilateral GPi can be tried.

In suspected autoimmune encephalitis, immunotherapy should be initiated as early as possible for the best recovery. Further management of autoimmune encephalitis is discussed elsewhere in this book.

Oral or nasogastric medications are avoided in any emergency due to erratic absorption. If the drugs are available only in the oral form, rapidly acting formulations are preferred.

Surgical intervention for movement disorder emergencies is slowly gaining popularity. DBS of bilateral GPi is now considered in dystonic storm soon after initial stabilization. This is especially useful if the patient has an underlying *DYT1* mutation. The DBS can be life-saving in this condition, since they can rapidly terminate the storm.

Immunotherapy is recommended if an autoimmune etiology is suspected, such as anti-NMDAR encephalitis, anti-LGI1 encephalitis, etc. Rapid initiation of IV methylprednisolone and/or immunoglobulins is associated with a good outcome.

Subacute Management

Postinitial stabilization, these conditions require disease-specific strategies to avoid recurrence of the emergency. General strategies during this period include:

- Antibiotic administration till resolution of any underlying infection
- Switch parenteral medications to oral medications.

Neuroleptic malignant syndrome:

- Stop all neuroleptics for 2 weeks.
- Restart at a low dose with gradual titration.
- Use low potency of neuroleptics.

Serotonergic syndrome:

- Monitor till washout of offending drug.

Dystonic storm:

- Treat any underlying precipitating infection.
- Avoid sudden withdrawal of any antidystonic medication.
- *Trials of oral medications*:
    - Trihexiphenidyl 3–6 mg/day initial dose
    - Risperidone 2–6 mg daily
    - Sulpiride 200–800 mg/day
    - Tetrabenazine 12.5–100 mg/day
    - Clonidine, clonazepam, and baclofen
- Consider baclofen, benzodiazepines, or levodopa

Acute dystonic reaction:

- Reassure the patient that this reaction is self-limiting and will wear off.
- Follow IV anticholinergics with oral maintenance for 7 days.
- Benzodiazepines can be useful in milder cases.
- Prophylactic use of anticholinergics or amantadine has not been found to be beneficial and is not recommended.

CONCLUSION

Emergencies in movement disorders represent conditions where rapid assessment and management can make a big difference in clinical outcomes and quality of life. Recognizing the phenomenology and establishing the syndrome are critical to this process.

REFERENCES

1. Rajan S, Kaas B, Moukheiber E. Movement disorders emergencies. In: McArthur JC, Stitt D (Eds). Seminars in neurology. New York: Thieme Medical Publishers; 2019. pp. 125-36.
2. Munhoz RP, Scorr LM, Factor SA. Movement disorders emergencies. Curr Opin Neurol. 2015;28(4):406-12.
3. Bhoyar A, Mahale R, Kamble N, Holla V, Pal P, Yadav R. Spectrum of movement disorder emergencies in a tertiary care center in India: A prospective observational study. Ann Indian Acad Neurol. 2022;25(5):890.
4. Kirkham FJ, Haywood P, Kashyape P, Borbone J, Lording A, Pryde K, et al. Movement disorder emergencies in childhood. Eur J Paediatr Neurol. 2011;15(5):390-404.
5. Ganti L, Rosario J. Movement Disorder Emergencies. In: Ganti L, Goldstein JN (eds). Neurologic Emergencies [Internet]. Cham: Springer International Publishing; 2018 [cited 2024 May 28]. pp. 271-87.
6. Gandhi SE, Newman EJ, Marshall VL. Emergency presentations of movement disorders. Pract Neurol. 2020;20(4):practneurol-2019-002277.
7. Frucht SJ. Movement disorder emergencies: diagnosis and treatment, Third edition. Cham, Switzerland: Humana Press; 2022.
8. Dalakas MC. Therapies in stiff-person syndrome: advances and future prospects based on disease pathophysiology. Neurology: Neuroimmunol Neuroinflam. 2023;10(3):e200109.
9. Cossu G. Hyperkinetic Movement Disorder Emergencies. Curr Neurol Neurosci Rep. 2017; 17(1):6.
10. Ali F, Wijdicks EF. Treatment of Movement Disorder Emergencies in Autoimmune Encephalitis in the Neurosciences ICU. Neurocrit Care. 2020;32(1): 286-94.

CHAPTER 13

Treatable Movement Disorders: Wilson Disease and Beyond

Vishwakiran Jhawar, Kuldeep Shetty, Prashanth LK

ABSTRACT

This chapter provides a comprehensive overview of treatable movement disorders, encompassing both hyperkinetic and hypokinetic conditions. We explore a range of etiologies, including metabolic, drug-induced, functional, autoimmune, infectious, and genetic causes, highlighting the potential for significant clinical improvement or complete cure through targeted treatments. The discussion begins with hyperkinetic disorders, detailing autoimmune and paraneoplastic diseases, infectious causes, acute metabolic disorders, drug-induced conditions, and treatable genetic diseases. We then examine hypokinetic disorders, focusing on parkinsonism and stiff person syndrome, elucidating their diverse etiologies and treatment approaches. A dedicated section on Wilson disease emphasizes the combination of tremor, dystonia, and parkinsonism, alongside diagnostic and therapeutic strategies. The chapter concludes with a review of various interventions, including botulinum toxin, deep brain stimulation (DBS), lesional surgeries, and other advanced treatments. Emphasizing the importance of identifying reversible causes, this chapter underscores the role of pathogenic and symptomatic treatments in improving patient outcomes and quality of life. Ongoing research and advancements continue to offer hope for those affected by these complex disorders.

Keywords: Treatment, Reversible movement disorders, Wilson's disease, Autoimmune movement disorders.

INTRODUCTION

Movement disorders encompass a range of conditions characterized by abnormal voluntary or involuntary movements, categorized into hypokinetic and hyperkinetic disorders. These disorders can arise from various etiologies such as metabolic, drug-induced, functional, autoimmune, infectious, and genetic causes. Importantly, many of these disorders are either fully curable or can be significantly improved through pathogenic or symptomatic treatments.[1] In this chapter, we systematically explore treatable movement disorders by initially describing hyperkinetic disorders based on their etiology due to the diverse clinical phenotypes they encompass, followed by an examination of hypokinetic disorders, categorized phenotype-wise given their limited clinical presentations **(Fig. 1)**. We also offer focused insights into Wilson disease and functional movement disorders and conclude by discussing various therapeutic interventions including botulinum toxin, deep brain stimulation (DBS), lesional surgeries, and other treatment approaches.

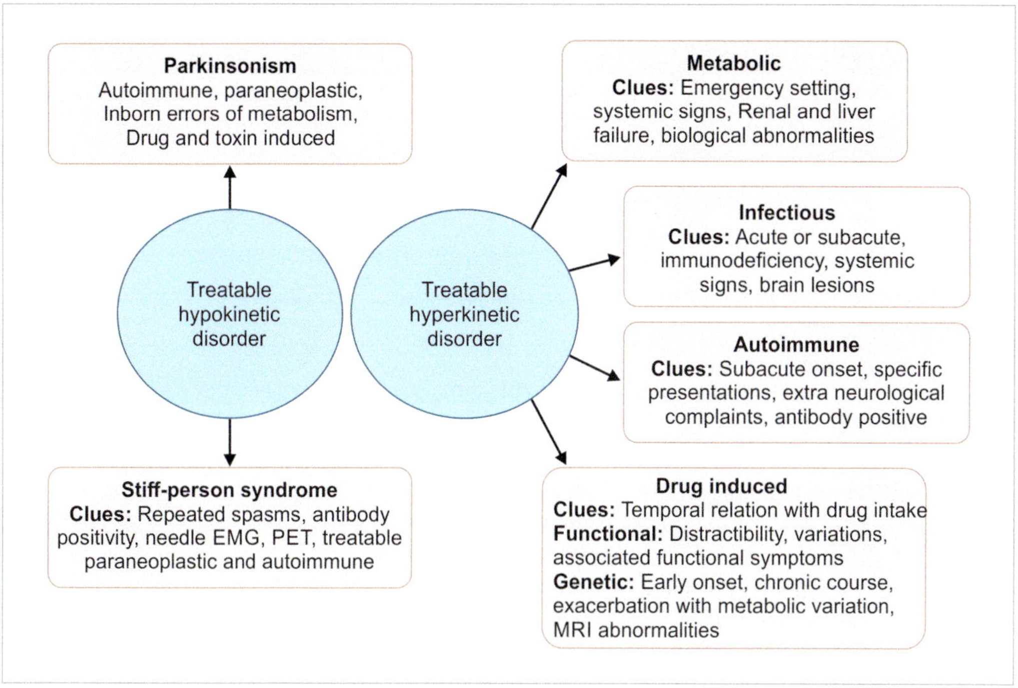

FIG. 1: Overview and clues for treatable movement disorders.

HYPERKINETIC DISORDERS

Autoimmune and Paraneoplastic Diseases (Table 1)[2,3]

- *Leucine-rich-glioma-inactivated (LGI) encephalitis*: Presents with stereotyped faciobrachial seizures, myoclonus, chorea, and parkinsonism, often accompanied by hyponatremia and rapid eye movement (REM) sleep behavior disorder. MRI typically reveals features of limbic encephalitis, and cerebrospinal fluid (CSF) shows pleocytosis. The most common associated tumor is thymoma. Treatment with immunomodulatory therapy often results in substantial clinical improvement.
- *Anti-Caspr-2 encephalitis*: Associated with neuromyotonia, chorea, ataxia, orthostatic myoclonus syndrome, Morvan syndrome, and limbic encephalitis. The disease course is usually slower compared to others, and most patients respond to immunomodulators.
- *Anti-N-methyl-D-aspartate (NMDA) receptor encephalitis*: Presents with orofacial dyskinesia, catatonia, limb dystonia, stereotypies, chorea, amnesia, psychiatric features, seizures, dysautonomia, and coma. Often associated with ovarian teratoma. Electroencephalography (EEG) shows extreme delta brush activity, CSF shows pleocytosis, MRI may be normal or show transient abnormalities in cortical or subcortical structures, and positron emission tomography (PET) reveals increased metabolism in the frontal and occipital regions. Diagnosis is confirmed with antibody tests against the GluN1 subunit of the NMDA receptor. Treatment includes immunomodulation with intravenous methylprednisolone (IVMP) and immunoglobulin (IVIG).

TABLE 1: Immune-mediated movement disorders

Cause	Movement disorders	Laboratory testing	MRI brain	Treatment
Antiphospholipid syndrome	• Chorea++ • PNKD, myoclonus, dystonia, and ataxia	APLA profile	Normal/ Ischemic stroke	Antithrombotic therapy
Lupus	Chorea, PNKD, myoclonus, dystonia, and ataxia	ANA profile	Normal	Immunotherapy
Anti-NMDA encephalitis	Orofacial dyskinesia, chorea, dystonia, and myoclonus	Autoimmune panel	Possible T2 hyperintensities	Immunotherapy
Anti-LGI1 encephalitis	Faciobrachial dystonic seizures	Anti-LGI1 antibodies	Possible T2 hyperintensities	Immunotherapy
Anti-IgLONS disease	Chorea, myoclonus, and ataxia	Anti-IgLON5 antibodies, polysomnography abnormalities, and central hypoventilation	Normal or brain atrophy	Immunotherapy
Celiac disease	Chorea, myoclonus, restless legs syndrome, dystonia, tremor, paroxysmal dyskinesia, and ataxia	Anti-transglutaminase and/or anti-gliadin antibodies, and positive duodenal biopsy		Immunotherapy
Hashimoto's encephalopathy	Myoclonus, dystonia, tremor, and chorea	Anti-Ig and anti-TPO antibodies, and possible thyroiditis	Possible T2 hyperintensities	Immunotherapy
Anti-CV2/CRMP-5, anti-D2R, anti-Hu encephalitis	Chorea	Anti-CV2/CRMP-5, anti-D2R, and anti-Hu antibodies	Possible basal ganglia T2 hyperintensities	Immunotherapy

(ANA: antinuclear antibody; APLA: antiphospholipid antibodies; CRMP-5: collapsin response mediator protein 5; D2R: dopamine receptor; LGI1: leucine-rich glioma-inactivated 1; NMDA: N-methyl-D-aspartate; PNKD: paroxysmal nonkinesigenic dyskinesia; TPO: thyroid peroxidase)

- *Anti-Yo and anti-Hu antibodies*: Found in ovarian and breast carcinoma, these antibodies are associated with significant cerebellar ataxia.
- *Antiglial fibrillary acidic protein (GFAP) antibodies*: Present with tremor, ataxia, encephalopathy, meningitis, myelopathy, seizures, dysautonomia, and psychiatric features, and may be seen in ovarian teratoma and prostate adenocarcinoma.
- *Anti-dipeptidyl-peptidase-like protein-6 (DPPX) antibodies*: Present with progressive encephalomyelitis with rigidity and myoclonus (PERM), opsoclonus-myoclonus syndrome (OMS), tremor, ataxia, behavioral changes, cognitive decline, seizures, dysautonomia, diarrhea, and weight loss, often seen in B-cell neoplasms.
- *Antineurexin-3-α-antibodies*: Associated with orofacial dyskinesias, confusion, seizures, and decreased level of consciousness.
- *Anticollapsing response-mediator protein-5 (CRMP-5)/CV2 encephalitis*: Presents with chorea, ataxia, opsoclonus-myoclonus syndrome (OMS), limbic encephalitis, encephalomyelitis, and

neuropathies, and may be associated with small cell lung carcinoma and thymoma.

Nonparaneoplastic Autoimmune Conditions[4]

- *Antiphospholipid syndrome (APS)*: Chorea is the most frequent manifestation.
- *Steroid-responsive encephalopathy associated with autoimmune thyroiditis (SREAT)*: Characterized by myoclonus, ataxia, and encephalopathy, diagnosed by the presence of antithyroid peroxidase (TPO) and antithyroglobulin (TG) antibodies.
- *Other conditions*: Include postinfectious encephalitis, celiac disease, and systemic lupus erythematosus (SLE).

Infectious Diseases

Infections affecting the basal ganglia can result from lesions, acute encephalitis, or delayed immune-mediated processes, causing up to 20% of secondary movement disorders **(Table 2)**.

- *Sydenham chorea*:[5] A major clinical manifestation of acute rheumatic fever caused by Group A streptococcal

TABLE 2: Neuroinfections and movement disorders.

Disease	Movement disorder	Investigation	Treatment
HIV	Chorea, tremor, myoclonus, dystonia, and paroxysmal dyskinesia	Serology, P24 antigen RT-PCR in serum and CSF	Highly active combination antiretroviral therapy with high penetrance in the central nervous system
Whipple disease	Oculomasticatory myorhythmia and oculofacioskeletal myorhythmia, and myoclonus	Tropheryma whipplei PCR in CSF, serum, saliva, feces PAS positivity on small bowel biopsy	Doxycycline 200 mg/day and hydroxychloroquine 600 mg/day for 12 months, followed by lifetime treatment with doxycycline 200 mg/day
Neurosyphilis	Chorea, myoclonus with cerebellar ataxia, and orofacial and/or laryngeal dystonia	Treponemal (TPHA) and nontreponemal (VDRL) tests in serum and CSF HIV serology, and brain MRI	• First line: Benzyl penicillin 18–24 million units IV daily (10–14 days) • Second line (if hospitalization and IV benzyl penicillin are impossible): • Ceftriaxone 1–2 g IV daily (10–14 days) • Procaine penicillin 1.2–2.4 million units IM daily and probenecid 500 mg QID (both 10–14 days)
Cryptococcus	Hemichorea-hemiballismus and myoclonus	Cryptococcal antigen (CRAG) detection and culture in serum and CSF, India ink staining of CSF	• Induction therapy (at least 2 weeks): Amphotericin B 3–4 mg/kg IV daily + flucytosine 25 mg/kg PO QID • Consolidation therapy (at least 8 weeks): Fluconazole 400 mg PO (or IV) daily • Maintenance therapy (at least 12 months): Fluconazole 200 mg PO daily

Continued

Continued

Disease	Movement disorder	Investigation	Treatment
Cysticercosis	Postural and kinetic tremor, EPC can be misdiagnosed as movement disorder	Serology in serum and CSF and PCR in CSF	Albendazole 15–30 mg/kg/day + praziquantel 50 mg/kg per day (15 days) + dexamethasone 0.1 mg/kg/day given 1–2 days before therapy
Sydenham chorea (SC) and PANDAS	Chorea and Tics (Motor and Ocular)	Throat swab for GAS rapid test and culture (patient and contacts) ASO	• Penicillin V PO (10 days): Children—250 mg/dose BID or TID; adolescents or adults—500 mg/dose BID or amoxicillin PO 10 days 50 mg/kg once daily, maximum 1 g • Chorea paralytica: Prednisone (2 mg/kg/day) or methylprednisolone (25 mg/kg/day) for 3–4 weeks SC refractory to antibiotic therapy: IVIG or plasmapheresis
Opsoclonus-myoclonus-ataxia syndrome	Myoclonus	Wide infectious assessment (HIV, HHV-6, CMV, West-Nile virus)	Antimicrobial therapy when appropriate immunotherapy: Corticosteroids, IVIG, or both

(ASO: antisense oligonucleotides; CSF: cerebrospinal fluid; GAS: group A *Streptococcus*; HIV: human immunodeficiency virus; IVIG: intravenous immunoglobulin; PANDAS: pediatric autoimmune neuropsychiatric disorder associated with group A streptococci; PAS: periodic acid-Schiff; RT-PCR: reverse transcription–polymerase chain reaction; TPHA: treponema pallidum hemagglutination; VDRL: The Venereal Disease Research Laboratory)

infection. Symptoms include chorea, motor impersistence, emotional changes, irritability, distractibility, and obsessive-compulsive symptoms. Psychiatric symptoms may include carditis. Diagnosis involves CSF analysis and MRI to exclude other causes. Treatment includes D2-receptor blockers, anti-seizure medications, steroids, and antibiotics. Most patients recover fully without treatment, with symptoms lasting from weeks to a year.

- *Whipple's disease:*[6] Caused by *Tropheryma whipplei,* characterized by oculomasticatory and oculofacioskeletal myorhythmia, often associated with altered mental status, cerebellar ataxia, tremor, dystonia, bruxism, chorea, and parkinsonism. Diagnosis includes MRI, EEG, small bowel biopsy, and CSF cytology. Treatment involves antibiotics.
- *Pediatric autoimmune neuropsychiatric disorder associated with group A streptococci (PANDAS):*[7] PANDAS presenting with obsessive-compulsive disorder (OCD), tic disorders, or other neuropsychiatric symptoms. Criteria include OCD and/or tic disorder, pediatric onset, abrupt onset, episodic course of symptoms, temporal relation with GAS infection, and tics during exacerbation. Treatment involves antistreptococcal antibiotics.

Acute Metabolic Disorders

- *Liver disease:*[8,9] Hepatic encephalopathy can cause myoclonus, tremor, chorea, and parkinsonism. MRI shows T1 hyperintensities in the internal pallidum and putamen, reversible with treatment. Mechanisms include toxic substance accumulation, altered neurotransmission, neuroinflammation, and stress. Treatment primarily involves hepatic transplantation, with ammonia-reducing therapy like lactulose improving some symptoms.

- *Renal disease:*[10] Uremic encephalopathy can cause stimulus-sensitive myoclonus and asterixis, improving with dialysis or renal transplant. Dialysis encephalopathy can result in myoclonus, dysarthria, and seizures due to aluminum poisoning or rapid uremia reduction. Treatment includes slowly correcting uremia and avoiding aluminum-containing dialysis solutions.
- *Blood sugar disturbance and dyselectrolytemia:*[11] Diabetic striatopathy is a hyperglycemic condition characterized by chorea/ballism and striatal hyperdensity, often in women with poorly controlled type 2 diabetes. Hypoglycemia episodes may cause mixed hyperkinetic movements, behavioral disturbances, and dysautonomia. Hypocalcemia can cause dystonia or carpopedal spasm, and hypomagnesemia can cause tremors, ataxia, and chorea. Hyperthyroidism can manifest as action or positional tremor and various hyperkinetic movements.[12] Vitamin B12 deficiency can cause chorea, tremor, and myoclonus.[13]

Drug-induced Hyperkinetic Movement Disorders

Drugs account for 3% of acute hyperkinetic movement disorders in children and 20% in adults over 50 years. These illnesses can be preventable or curable, with a correlation between drug introduction and movement occurrence suggesting a strong link.

- *Tardive syndromes:*[14,15] Caused by long-term exposure to dopamine receptor blockers, they include dyskinesia, dystonia, stereotypies, and more. Treatment involves dopamine depleting agents, vesicular monoamine transporter 2 (VMAT-2) inhibitors, botox, and GPi-DBS in refractory cases.

Treatable Genetic Diseases

Genetic diseases are rare causes of treatable hyperkinetic movement disorders, often indicated by onset in childhood or adolescence, family history, and chronic disease course. Examples include young-onset Parkinson's disease, juvenile Huntington's disease, and neurodegeneration with brain iron accumulation (NBIA) **(Table 3)**.

HYPOKINETIC DISORDERS

Hypokinetic disorders mainly comprise parkinsonism and stiff person syndrome due to various etiologies.

Parkinsonism

- *Systemic autoimmune disease*: Includes primary Sjögren syndrome, systemic lupus erythematosus (SLE), antiphospholipid syndrome (APS), and rheumatoid arthritis. Treatment involves immunomodulators and symptomatic treatments.
- *Autoimmune and paraneoplastic parkinsonism*: Includes disorders such as anti-IgLON-5, anti-Ma2, and anti-Ri-2 associated with various cancers and neurological symptoms, responsive to immunotherapy.
- *Genetic diseases*: Includes Parkinson's disease, Wilson disease, Huntington's disease, and NBIA, with specific genetic mutations identified and treatments varying from symptomatic relief to specific interventions like deferoxamine for NBIA.
- *Drug and toxin-induced parkinsonism*: Caused by antipsychotics,[16] antiemetics, dopamine depleting agents, and other medications,[17] as well as toxins such as carbon monoxide and manganese.

TABLE 3: Treatable Inheritable disorders.

Etiology	Movement disorders	Diagnostic cues	Laboratory findings	Treatment
Paroxysmal kinesigenic dyskinesia	• Isolated • Paroxysmal • Kinesigenic • Dyskinesia	–	*PRRT2* mutation	Antiepileptics (Na channel blockers)
SLC30A10- and *SLC39A14*-associated hyper-magnesemia	Dystonia, Parkinsonism spasticity	Hypermagnesemia and hepatic cirrhosis	MRI symmetric TI signal hyper-intensity in the basal ganglia consistent with manganese deposition	Chelation (disodium calcium EDTA)
ADCY5-related dyskinesia	Pleiotropic paroxysmal dyskinesia, orofacial myoclonus	Nocturnal episodes, hypotonia, and fluctuations	*ADCY5* mutation (possibly mosaic)	Caffeine
GLUT-1 deficiency	Paroxysmal exercise-induced dyskinesia, ataxia, and dystonia	Seizures, worsening with fasting or exercise	Low CSF glucose levels, *SLC2A1* mutation	Ketogenic diet Triheptanoin
DOPA responsive dystonia	Dystonia, paroxysmal exercise-induced dyskinesia	Motor fluctuations, sleep benefit, and oculogyric crises	Abnormal CSF neurotransmitters, *GCH1, TH, SPR*, or *PTPS* mutation	Levodopa
Glutaric aciduria type 1	Dystonia, parkinsonism, and chorea	Acute encephalopathy episodes	Elevated glutaric acid in plasma and/or urine, *GCDH* mutations	Low-lysine diet, carnitine supplementation
Pyruvate dehydrogenase deficiency	Dystonia and paroxysmal dystonia	Episodic ataxia Bi-pallidal lesions on MR	High lactate and pyruvate levels, *PDHA1, PDHA2, PDHX*, or *DLAT* mutations	Thiamine ketogenic diet
Niemann–Pick disease C	Dystonia, chorea, myoclonus, and parkinsonism	Ataxia and supranuclear gaze palsy	Elevated serum oxysterols, *NPC1* or *NPC2* mutations	Miglustat
AVED (Ataxia with vitamin E deficiency)	Dystonia and head tremor	Ataxia	Very low plasma vitamin E and *TTPA* mutations	High doses of vitamin E

Continued

Continued

Etiology	Movement disorders	Diagnostic cues	Laboratory findings	Treatment
Cerebrotendinous xanthomatosis	Ataxia, spasticity, and parkinsonism	Chronic diarrhea and early cataract	High plasma cholestanol and *CYP27A1* mutations	Chenodeoxycholic acid
Segawa disease (GTPCH deficiency)	Dystonia, postural tremor, and parkinsonism	Depression, anxiety, and spastic diplegia	CSF neurotrans-mitter levels, phenylalanine load test, L-DOPA trial, *GCH1* sequencing	Levodopa/ Carbidopa
Biotin and thiamine responsive basal ganglia disease	Dystonia, parkinsonism, and ataxia spasticity	Subacute encephalopathy, dysarthria, dysphagia, external ophthalmoplegia, and seizures	Brain MRI and *SLC19A3* sequencing	Treatment: thiamine and biotin

(CSF: cerebrospinal fluid; DOPA: dihydroxyphenylalanine; EDTA: ethylenediaminetetraacetic acid; GTPCH: guanosine triphosphate cyclohydrolase; PTPS: pyruvoyl tetrahydropterin synthase)

- *Infectious diseases*: Includes chronic viral encephalitis, West Nile virus, Japanese encephalitis, human immunodeficiency virus (HIV)/acquired immunodeficiency syndrome (AIDS), neurosyphilis, prion disease, and progressive multifocal leukoencephalopathy, with treatment focused on the underlying infection and symptomatic relief.[18]
- *Metabolic conditions*: Includes Fahr's disease[19] and other metabolic disorders, with treatment involving managing underlying metabolic abnormalities.
- *Normal pressure hydrocephalus (NPH)*: Diagnosed by gait disturbance, cognitive decline, and urinary incontinence, with treatment often involving ventriculo-peritoneal (VP) shunting.[20]

Stiff-person Syndrome

Characterized by fluctuating muscle rigidity and spasms, often misdiagnosed as functional disorders. Associated antibodies include anti-glutamic acid decarboxylase (GAD), glycine receptor antibodies, and others. Treatment includes symptomatic medications such as diazepam and baclofen, antiepileptics, and immunomodulators.[21]

WILSON DISEASE

Wilson disease presents with a combination of tremor, dystonia, and parkinsonism, often characterized by wing-beating tremor and orofacial involvement. Diagnosis involves copper levels in serum and liver, serum ceruloplasmin levels, MRI, and genetic testing. Treatment includes chelating agents and zinc therapy **(Table 4)**.[22,23]

INTERVENTIONS IN MOVEMENT DISORDERS

- *Botulinum toxin*: Although primarily symptomatic, sustained use significantly improves quality of life, often resulting in near-total symptom resolution.[24]

TABLE 4: Decoppering therapy for Wilson disease.

Drug	Mode of action	Neurological worsening	Side effects	Comments	Dose
D-penicil-lamine	Chelator induces renal excretion of copper	10–20% during initial phase	Fever/Rash/Bone marrow suppression/ Hepatotoxicity/Colitis/ Serous retinitis	Reduce dose during pregnancy and during surgery	1 g/day (0.5–2.0 g/day) before food with pyridoxine 25 mg/day
Zinc	Metallothionein inducer, and blocks intestinal copper absorption	Can occur during initial phase of treatment	Gastritis and biochemical pancreatitis	No dosage reduction in pregnancy and during surgery	50–200 mg three times per day
Trientene	Chelator induces renal excretion of copper	10–15% during initial phase	Gastritis, aplastic anemia, sideroblastic anemia, and colitis	Reduce dose during pregnancy and during surgery	1–2 g/day (250–500 mg four times per day)

- *Deep brain stimulation and lesional procedures*: DBS provides sustained symptomatic benefits, especially in Parkinson's disease and dystonia, with specific indications for use.[25]
- *Lesional surgeries*: Thalamotomy, pallidotomy, and partial thromboplastin time (PTT) lesions offer cost-effective alternatives to DBS, especially when performed unilaterally.
- *Other interventions*: Includes baclofen pumps,[26] Levodopa carbidopa intestinal gel,[27] apomorphine pumps,[28] and selective dorsal rhizotomy,[29] each providing specific benefits in managing movement disorders.

CONCLUSION

Movement disorders are a diverse group of conditions characterized by abnormal voluntary or involuntary movements. Identifying and investigating reversible causes is crucial in the management of these disorders. A thorough assessment should consider the temporal correlation between the onset of symptoms and drug intake, as this can provide significant diagnostic clues. Recognizing the specific type of movement disorder is essential for narrowing down the diagnosis and formulating an effective treatment plan. Treatment strategies often involve addressing the underlying causes, utilizing immunomodulation, dietary changes, nutritional replacement, and antibiotics as necessary. Symptomatic treatments play a pivotal role in patient management and include medications such as levodopa, anticholinergics, botulinum toxin, as well as advanced interventions like DBS and lesional therapies.

In conclusion, understanding the etiology and clinical manifestations of movement disorders enables clinicians to implement targeted and effective therapeutic interventions. By combining pathogenic treatments with symptomatic relief strategies, significant improvements in patient's outcomes and quality of life can be achieved. Ongoing research and advancements in treatment modalities continue to offer hope for those affected by these complex and challenging disorders.

REFERENCES

1. Menozzi E, Mulroy E, Akbarian-Tefaghi L, Bhatia KP, Balint B. Movement disorders in systemic autoimmune diseases: Clinical spectrum, ancillary investigations, pathophysiological considerations. Parkinsonism Relat Disord [Internet]. 2021;88:116-28.
2. Damato V, Balint B, Kienzler AK, Irani SR. The clinical features, underlying immunology, and treatment of autoantibody-mediated movement disorders. Mov Disord [Internet]. 2018;33(9):1376-89.
3. Chirra M, Marsili L, Gallerini S, Keeling EG, Marconi R, Colosimo C. Paraneoplastic movement disorders: phenomenology, diagnosis, and treatment. Eur J Intern Med [Internet]. 2019;67:14-23.
4. Chorea SS. Original articles. Eur J Gen Pract. 2006;12(1):1.
5. Zomorrodi A, Wald ER. Sydenham's chorea in western Pennsylvania. Pediatrics [Internet]. 2006;117(4):e675-9.
6. Bally JF, Méneret A, Roze E, Anderson M, Grabli D, Lang AE. Systematic review of movement disorders and oculomotor abnormalities in Whipple's disease. Mov Disord [Internet]. 2018;33(11):1700-11.
7. Swedo SE, Leonard HL, Garvey M, Mittleman B, Allen AJ, Perlmutter S, et al. Pediatric Autoimmune Neuropsychiatric Disorders Associated With Streptococcal Infections: Clinical Description of the First 50 Cases. Am J Psychiatry [Internet]. 1998;155(2):264-71.
8. Sousa AL, Salgado P, Alves JE, Silva S, Ferreira S, Magalhães M. Uncommon Movement Disorders in Chronic Hepatic Disease with Response to Rifaximin. Tremor Other Hyperkinet Mov (N Y) [Internet]. 2019;9.
9. Shin HW, Park HK. Recent Updates on Acquired Hepatocerebral Degeneration. Tremor Other Hyperkinet Mov (N Y) [Internet]. 2017;7:463.
10. Eberhardt O, Topka H. Myoclonic Disorders. Brain Sci [Internet]. 2017;7(8):103.
11. Dizon AM, Kowalyk S, Hoogwerf BJ. Neuroglycopenic and other symptoms in patients with insulinomas. Am J Med [Internet]. 1999;106(3):307-10.
12. Tan EK, Chan LL. Movement disorders associated with hyperthyroidism: expanding the phenotype. Mov Disord [Internet]. 2006;21(7):1054-5.
13. de Souza A, Moloi MW. Involuntary movements due to vitamin B12 deficiency. Neurol Res [Internet]. 2014;36(12):1121-8.
14. Estevez-Fraga C, Zeun P, López-Sendón Moreno JL. Current Methods for the Treatment and Prevention of Drug-Induced Parkinsonism and Tardive Dyskinesia in the Elderly. Drugs Aging [Internet]. 2018;35(11):959-71.
15. Frei K, Truong DD, Fahn S, Jankovic J, Hauser RA. The nosology of tardive syndromes. J Neurol Sci [Internet]. 2018;389:10-6.
16. Rochon PA, Stukel TA, Sykora K, Gill S, Garfinkel S, Anderson GM, et al. Atypical Antipsychotics and Parkinsonism. Arch Intern Med [Internet]. 2005;165(16):1882.
17. Faber R, Trimble MR. Electroconvulsive therapy in Parkinson's disease and other movement disorders. Mov Disord [Internet]. 1991;6(4):293-303.
18. Leta V, Urso D, Batzu L, Lau YH, Mathew D, Boura I, et al. Viruses, parkinsonism and Parkinson's disease: the past, present and future. J Neural Transm [Internet]. 2022;129(9):1119-32.
19. Saleem S, Aslam HM, Anwar M, Anwar S, Saleem M, Saleem A, et al. Fahr's syndrome: literature review of current evidence. Orphanet J Rare Dis [Internet]. 2013;8(1):156.
20. Jankovic J, Tolosa E. Parkinson's disease and movement disorders Philadelphia, PA: Lippincott Williams & Wilkins; 2002. pp. 473-82.
21. Baizabal-Carvallo JF, Jankovic J. Stiff-person syndrome: Insights into a complex autoimmune disorder. J Neurol Neurosurg Psychiatry. 2015;86(8):840-8.
22. Nagral A, Sarma MS, Matthai J, Kukkle PL, Devarbhavi H, Sinha S, et al. Wilson's Disease: Clinical Practice Guidelines of the Indian National Association for Study of the Liver, the Indian Society of Pediatric Gastroenterology, Hepatology and Nutrition, and the Movement Disorders Society of India. J Clin Exp Hepatol. 2019;9(1):74-98.
23. Factor SA, Podskalny GD, Molho ES. Psychogenic movement disorders: frequency, clinical profile, and characteristics. J Neurol Neurosurg Psychiatry [Internet]. 1995;59(4):406-12.
24. Jankovic J. Botulinum toxin: State of the art. Mov Disord [Internet]. 2017;32(8):1131-8.
25. Kaelin-Lang A, You H, Burgunder JM, Lönnfors-Weitze T, Loher TJ, Taub E, et al. Bilateral pallidal stimulation improves cervical dystonia for more than a decade. Parkinsonism Relat Disord [Internet]. 2020;81:78-81.

26. Motta F, Buonaguro V, Stignani C. The use of intrathecal baclofen pump implants in children and adolescents: safety and complications in 200 consecutive cases. J Neurosurg [Internet]. 2007;107(1 Suppl):32-5.
27. Thakkar S, Fung VSC, Merola A, Rollins M, Soileau MJ, Kovács N. 24-Hour Levodopa-Carbidopa Intestinal Gel: Clinical Experience and Practical Recommendations. CNS Drugs [Internet]. 2021;35(2):137-49.
28. Brinker D, Smilowska K, Paschen S, Antonini A, Moro E, Deuschl G. How to Use the New European Academy of Neurology/Movement Disorder Society European Section Guideline for Invasive Therapies in Parkinson's Disease. Mov Disord Clin Pract [Internet]. 2024;11(3):209-19.
29. Abou Al-Shaar H, Imtiaz MT, Alhalabi H, Alsubaie SM, Sabbagh AJ. Selective dorsal rhizotomy: A multidisciplinary approach to treating spastic diplegia. Asian J Neurosurg [Internet]. 2017;12(3):454-65.

Index

Page numbers followed by *b* refer to box, *f* refer to figure, *fc* refer to flowchart, and *t* refer to table.

C

H

I

J

K

L

T